Hemendra Kumar Sharma
Sandhya Chaurasia
Suneel Kumar Vasireddy

Formulation and Evaluation of Cephalexin Extended Release Tablet

Hemendra Kumar Sharma
Sandhya Chaurasia
Suneel Kumar Vasireddy

Formulation and Evaluation of Cephalexin Extended Release Tablet

Comparatively Study with Marketed Formulations

LAP LAMBERT Academic Publishing

Impressum/Imprint (nur für Deutschland/only for Germany)
Bibliografische Information der Deutschen Nationalbibliothek: Die Deutsche Nationalbibliothek verzeichnet diese Publikation in der Deutschen Nationalbibliografie; detaillierte bibliografische Daten sind im Internet über http://dnb.d-nb.de abrufbar.
Alle in diesem Buch genannten Marken und Produktnamen unterliegen warenzeichen-, marken- oder patentrechtlichem Schutz bzw. sind Warenzeichen oder eingetragene Warenzeichen der jeweiligen Inhaber. Die Wiedergabe von Marken, Produktnamen, Gebrauchsnamen, Handelsnamen, Warenbezeichnungen u.s.w. in diesem Werk berechtigt auch ohne besondere Kennzeichnung nicht zu der Annahme, dass solche Namen im Sinne der Warenzeichen- und Markenschutzgesetzgebung als frei zu betrachten wären und daher von jedermann benutzt werden dürften.

Coverbild: www.ingimage.com

Verlag: LAP LAMBERT Academic Publishing GmbH & Co. KG
Heinrich-Böcking-Str. 6-8, 66121 Saarbrücken, Deutschland
Telefon +49 681 3720-310, Telefax +49 681 3720-3109
Email: info@lap-publishing.com

Approved by: *Sagar Institute of Research and Technology-Pharmacy Ayodhya By-Pass Road, Bhopal (M.P.)-462 041, India, RGPV University

Herstellung in Deutschland:
Schaltungsdienst Lange o.H.G., Berlin
Books on Demand GmbH, Norderstedt
Reha GmbH, Saarbrücken
Amazon Distribution GmbH, Leipzig
ISBN: 978-3-8484-3263-9

Imprint (only for USA, GB)
Bibliographic information published by the Deutsche Nationalbibliothek: The Deutsche Nationalbibliothek lists this publication in the Deutsche Nationalbibliografie; detailed bibliographic data are available in the Internet at http://dnb.d-nb.de.
Any brand names and product names mentioned in this book are subject to trademark, brand or patent protection and are trademarks or registered trademarks of their respective holders. The use of brand names, product names, common names, trade names, product descriptions etc. even without a particular marking in this works is in no way to be construed to mean that such names may be regarded as unrestricted in respect of trademark and brand protection legislation and could thus be used by anyone.

Cover image: www.ingimage.com

Publisher: LAP LAMBERT Academic Publishing GmbH & Co. KG
Heinrich-Böcking-Str. 6-8, 66121 Saarbrücken, Germany
Phone +49 681 3720-310, Fax +49 681 3720-3109
Email: info@lap-publishing.com

Printed in the U.S.A.
Printed in the U.K. by (see last page)
ISBN: 978-3-8484-3263-9

Index

Objectives

The novel design of an oral controlled drug delivery system should be primarily aimed at achieving more predictable and increased bioavailability of drugs. But there are several physiological difficulties, which include restraining and localizing the drug delivery system within the regions of the gastrointestinal tract and the highly variable nature of gastric emptyig process (a few minutes to 12 hours). This variability, in turn may lead to unpredictable bioavailability and the time to achieve peak plasma levels, since the majority of drugs are preferentially absorbed from the upper part of small intestine. Fruthermore, the relatively brief gastric emptying time in humans, which normally averages 2 to 3 hours through the major absorption zone (stomach or upper part of the intestine), can result in incomplete drug release from the drug delivery system leading to diminished efficacy of the administered dose. Therefore, restraining a drug delivery system in a specific region of the gastrointestinal tract offers numerous advantages, especially for drugs exhibiting an absorption window or for drugs with a stability problem. Overall, the intimate contact of the drug delivery system with the absorbing membrane has the potential to maximize drug absorption and may also influence the rate of drug absorption. These considerations have led to the development of oral controlled-release dosage forms possessing gastric retention capabilities. Various types of drugs, which can benefit from using gastroretentive devices are (a) drugs acting locally and primarily absorbed in the stomach, (b) drugs that are poorly soluble at an alkaline pH, (c) those with a narrow window of absorption, (d) drugs absorbed rapidly from the GI tract, and (e) drugs that degrade in the colon. Cephalexin is a semi-synthetic antibiotics used in the treatment of bacterial infection. It is completely absorbed from the gastrointestinal tract and has an oral bioavailability of only 90%, while the remaining is excreted unchanged in faeces. This is because of its poor absorption in lower gastrointestinal tract. It undergoes little or no hepatic first pass metabolism and its elimination half-life is 8 to 9 hours. Therefore, it is selected as a suitable drug for the design of a Extended release tablets with a view to improve its oral bioavailability. In the present work, an attempt has been made to formulate Extended release tablets of Cephalexin using hydroxy propyl methyl cellulose of different viscosity grades in order to prolong the drug release, and to impart floating properties to the matrix tablet formulations. After preliminary studies, optimization of designed ERT will be performed using direct compression methods. The validity of the derived polynomial equations for the dependent variables (dissolution parameters) will be verified by designing and evaluating two extra check point formulations.

Abstract

In this study, controlled release matrix tablets containing cephelexin were prepared using HPMC15 cps and Eudragit L100 in different concentration by Direct compression method. Tablets were evaluated for physical properties,Hardness, friability, weight variation and In vitro dissolution study was carried on USP II apparetus (peddle type). The best formulations selected based on above parameters were subjected for Extend release study with use of different ratio of polymer as Eudragit and HPMC .The tablets with Eudragit were found to release drug for longer duration of time as compared to formulations containing HPMC. The drug release from the tablets was sufficiently sustained.

Chapter-1

Introduction

Oral route has been the most commonly adopted and the most convenient route for drug delivery. Oral route of administration has received more attention in the pharmaceutical field because of more flexibility in the designing of dosage form than the drug delivery design for other routes (Vyas SP, 2002).

An ideal dosage regimen in the drug therapy of any disease is the one which immediately attains the desired therapeutic concentration of drug in plasma or at the site of action and maintains it constant for the entire duration of treatment. But since it is difficult to get both these features in normal conventional formulation, (Brahmankar DM, 1995) in last two decades the drug delivery technology has been developed rapidly and many novel oral drug delivery systems have been invented, and they are very helpful in achieving this goal of ideal dosage regimen. Novel oral drug delivery system has been broadly classified into two categories.

- Systemic Release Dosage Forms

- Drug Targeting Dosage Forms

The former system releases the drug in a controlled or modified manner in the GIT for systemic uptake with no particular area of GIT specified. While the later targets the drug to a specified part of body.

For formulation of FDC we usually desire that the dosage regimen should be designed in such a way so that the patient gets maximum benefit of the therapy without much strain. Direct tabletting of pharmaceutical materials is desirable to reduce the cost of production (Shangraw *et al.*, 1989). To succeed in direct compression, particle modification of a drug is required to impart the formula sufficient flowability and compressibility. The preparation of spherical agglomerates has come into the forefront of interest because the habit of the particles (form, shape, particle size distribution, surface, etc.) can be changed by the crystallization process (Szabo-Revesz *et al.*, 2001). The spherical crystallization is an efficient technique for particle design for direct tabletting, during which crystallization and agglomeration can be carried out in one-step. The physical properties of the agglomerated crystals can be controlled simultaneously without using any filler or binder. Spherical crystallization can be achieved by various methods such as spherical agglomeration, emulsion solvent diffusion, ammonia diffusion, and neutralization methods .Hence it is preferred that the FDCs are formulated as extended release formulations to reduce the dosage regimen.

1.1. Advantages of controlled release preparations: [4, 5]

Controlled release drug products offer several important advantages over immediate release conventional dosage form of the same drug.

1). More efficient drug utilization by the body.
2). Better patient compliance.
3). Decrease in frequency of administration.
4). Elimination of peak and valley plasma levels so that drug concentration is maintained
5) Constant over a long period of time. Hence reduction in severity and frequency of
6) Untoward side effects.
7). Safety margin of potent drug is increased.
8). Avoidance of nighttime dosing.
9). Reduction in GIT irritation and other dose related side effects.

1.2 Limitations of controlled release preparations: [2, 6]

1. Over dose: There is always the possibility of sudden release of the total dose administered i.e. dose dumping, which may result in some toxic manifestations.

2. Less flexibility in dose adjustments: It is very difficult to adjust the dose of control release products to a patient's response.

3. The physician has been less flexibility in adjusting the dosage regimens.

4. Side effects: Controlled release preparations would show not only a longer duration of effect but also a long duration of side effects, especially if the patient is hypersensitive to the given medication.

5. The cost of unit dose of controlled therapeutic system is higher than the regular conventional dosage forms.

6. Special treatment problems may arise during accidental poisoning with these systems.

7. Unpredictable and often poor '*In vitro-In vivo*' correlation.

8. More rapid development of tolerance to the drug.

1.3. Absorption Sites of Gastrointestinal Tract:
1.3.1 Stomach [7,8]

The main function of stomach is to store food temporarily, grind it and then release it slowly into the duodenum. The stomach is an important site of enzyme production. Due to its small surface area, very little absorption takes place from the stomach. It provides a barrier for the delivery of drugs to the small intestine. Anatomically stomach is divided into four regions namely, fundus, body, antrum, and pylorus. The main function of fundus and body is storage whereas that of antrum is mixing or grinding. The fundus adjusts to the increased volume during eating by relaxation of the fundal muscle fibers. The fundus also exerts a steady pressure on the gastric contents, pressing them towards the distal stomach. To pass through the pyloric valve into the small intestine, particles should be of the order of 1-2 mm. The antrum does this grinding. The stomach has limitation of short residence time.

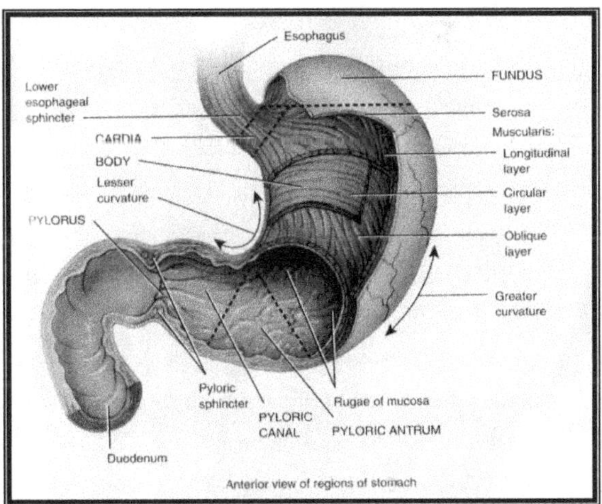

Figure 1- Internal Structure of human Stomach

1.3.2 Small Intestine

The small intestine is divided in to three parts, the first 20-30 cm is termed the duodenum, and the second 2.5 meters the jejunum and the final 3.5 meter the ileum. The main functions are to mix food with enzymes to facilitate digestion and circulate the intestinal contents with the intestinal secretions to enable absorption to occur and propel the unabsorbed materials in an above direction.

a) Absorption of drugs:

The principal permeability barrier is represented by the luminal surface of the brush border. Most of the drugs are absorbed by passive diffusion in their unionized state. The pH of the small intestine determines the degree of ionization and hence controls the efficiency of absorption, which is the basis of the pH partition theory of drug absorption. Protein binding at the serosal side of the epithelium helps to maintain a concentration gradient by binding the absorbed drug, which is then removed by blood flow from the absorption site.

b) Factors:

❖ **pH.**

The pH of small intestine determines the degree of ionization and hence controls the efficiency of absorption. The luminal pH is approximately 7, suggests that some acidic drugs such as salicylate, would not be well absorbed.

❖ **Interaction with food.**

The presence of food may influence the absorption of several drugs and can either enhance, delay or reduce absorption. The absorption of drugs such as penicillin V and G, Theophylline and Erythromycin is reduced by the presence of food, but food delays absorption of drugs such as Cimetidine, Metronidazole and Digoxin. Certain components of food, notably fiber, have a particularly important effect on drug absorption. Fiber is known to inhibit the absorption of Digoxin and entrap steroids. Several indirect methods have been employed to increase the contact time of a drug with the small intestinal surface, such as retention of the dosage form within the stomach, which then trickles drug over the absorptive surface.

1.3.3 Colon [9]

The colon forms the lower part of the gastrointestinal tract and extends from the ileocecal junction to the anus. The colon is upper 5 feet of the large intestine and the rectum is the lower 6 inches. While the colon is mainly situated in the abdomen, the rectum is primarily a pelvic organ. The colon is a cylindrical tube, which is lined by the moist, soft pink lining, called as mucosa; the pathway is called the lumen and is approximately 2-3 inches in diameter. The major function of the colon is the consolidation of the intestinal content into fasces by the absorption of water and electrolytes and to store the fasces until excretion.

1.3.3 (a) Absorption of drugs from the colon:

Drugs are absorbed passively by paracellular or transcellular routes. Transcellular absorption involves the passage of drugs through cells and this is the route most lipophilic drugs takes, where as paracellular absorption involves the transport of drug through the tight junctions between cells and is the route most hydrophilic drug takes. Studies in the rat have indicated that paracellular absorption is constant through small intestine, but transcellular absorption appears to be confined to the small intestine, with negligible colonic absorption by these routes. The poor paracellular absorption of many drugs in the colon is due to the fact that epithelial cell junctions are very tight. The slow rate of transit in colon lets the drug stay in contact with mucosa for a longer period than in small intestine, which compensates the much lower surface area.

1.3.4 Factors affecting colonic transit time: [9]

- ❖ **pH.**

On entry into the colon, the pH drops of 6.4 ± 0.6. The pH in the mid colon is 6.6±0.8 and in the left colon 7 ± 0.7. There is a fall in pH on entry into the colon due to the presence of short chain fatty acids arising from bacterial fermentation of polysaccharides. For example lactose is fermented by the colonic bacteria to produce large amounts of lactic acid resulting in pH drop to about 5.

❖ **Presence of food.**

The presence of food generally increases gastric residence and in some cases with regular feeding, dosage forms have been shown to reside in the stomach for periods in excess of 12 hrs. The total time for transit tends to be highly variable and influenced by a number of factors such as diet, in particular dietary fiber content, mobility, stress, disease and drugs. Ingestion of food has been found to stimulate colonic activity in what is termed the gastrocolonic response.

1.3.5 Factors affecting gastric emptying time

❖ **pH:**

Environmental pH affects the performance of orally administered drugs. The pH of stomach in fasted condition is about 1.5-2 and in fed conditions it is usually 2 to 6. A large volume of water administered with oral dosage form changes the pH of stomach to pH of water initially. This change occurs because stomach does not have enough time to produce sufficient quantity of acid before emptying of liquid from the stomach.

❖ Volume:

The resting volume of stomach is about 25-52 ml. Gastric volume is important for dissolution of the dosage forms *In-vivo*. Meyer et al. conducted an experiment to study the effect of gastric fluid volume on absorption of controlled release Theophylline dosage form in human beings. During this experiment they measured the gastric fluid volume of each subject. They estimated the mean gastric fluid volume in normal and achlorhydric subjects. The mean volume recovered by gastric aspiration over three consecutive, 15-min time periods was 61+ 51ml in achlorhydric subjects and 98+38ml in normal subjects. Thus there is

such a large volume difference in gastric secretions that would significantly affect *In vivo* dissolution of drugs.

❖ Gastric mucosa:

Simple columnar epithelial cells line the entire mucosal surface of the stomach. Mucus, parietal, and peptic cells are present in the body of stomach. These cells are associated with different functions. The parietal cells secrete acid whereas the peptic cells secrete precursor for pepsin. The surface mucosal cells secrete the mucus and bicarbonate.

❖ **Gastric secretions:**

Acids, pepsin, gastrin, mucus and some other enzymes are the secretions of the stomach. Normal adults produce a basal secretion up to 60ml with approximately 4m mol of hydrogen ions every hour. Other potent stimulators of gastric acid are the hormone gastrin, peptides, amino acids and gastric distention.

❖ **Effect of food on gastric secretion and gastric emptying:**

Type of meal and its caloric content, volume, viscosity and co-administered drugs affect gastric secretions and gastric emptying time. The rate of emptying primarily depends on caloric contents of the ingested meal. It does not differ for proteins, fats and carbohydrates as long as their caloric contents are the same. Generally gastric emptying is slowed down because of increased acidity, osmolarity and calorific values.

❖ **Hormonal effect:**

Stress increases gastric emptying rate whereas depression slows it down. Generally females have slow gastric emptying rate than males. Age and obesity also affect gastric emptying.

❖ **Presence of food:**

Gastric emptying of dosage forms is different in fasted and fed conditions. Volume of liquid affects gastric emptying of liquids. Liquids empty exponentially that is the larger the volume the faster is the gastric emptying.

1.4 Gastro Retentive Drug Delivery System: [11]

Oral route of administration is the most important and convenient route for drug delivery. The benefits of long-term delivery technology have not been fully realized for dosage forms designed for oral administration. This is mainly due to the fact that the extent of drug absorption from GIT is determined by GI physiology, irrespective of the control release properties of the device. Although differential absorption from various regions of GI has been known for decades, only recently drug delivery systems have been designed to target drugs to differential regions of GIT. These include gastro retentive systems, delayed release systems and colon targeting.

Overall, the intimate contact of the DDS with the absorbing membrane has the potential to maximize drug absorption and may also influence the rate of drug absorption. These considerations have lead to the development of oral controlled release dosage forms possessing gastric retention capabilities. The real issue in the development of oral controlled release dosage form is not just to prolong the delivery of drugs for more than 12 hrs but also to prolong the presence of dosage forms in the stomach or somewhere in the upper small intestine. Dosage forms with prolonged gastric residence time (GRT), i.e. gastro remaining or gastro retentive dosage form (GRDF), will bring about new and important therapeutic options.

For instance, these will significantly extend the period of time over which drugs may be released, and thus prolong dosing intervals and increase patient compliance beyond the compliance level of existing controlled release dosage forms. GRDF will also greatly improve the pharmacotherapy of the stomach itself through local drug release leading to high drug concentrations at the gastric mucosa, which are sustained over a long period of time. For example, eradication of *Helicobacter pylori*, which requires the administration of various medications several times a day according to a complicated regimen and which frequently fails as a result of insufficient patient compliance, could perhaps be achieved more reliably using GRDF to administer smaller drug doses for fewer times.

Finally, GRDF will be used as carriers for drugs with so called absorption windows; these substances are taken up only from very specific sites of the gastrointestinal mucosa, often in a proximal region of the small intestine. Conventional controlled release dosage forms pass the absorption window while they still contain a large and rather undefined portion of the dose which is consequently lost for absorption. In contrast, an appropriate GRDF would slowly release the complete dose over its defined GRT and thus make it continuously available to the appropriate tissue regions for absorption. Need of gastro retention arises of two reasons [2].

To improve bioavailability of drugs such as Cyclosporine, Ciprofloxacin, Cefuroxime-axetil, Ranitidine etc., which are mainly absorbed from upper part of GIT and or get degraded in basic pH. For local action in case of pathologies of stomach.

1.4.1. Approaches for Gastric Retention: [11]

A. Floating System (Low Density Approach):

These systems are also known as hydro dynamically balanced systems. (HBS/FDDS) They have a bulk density lower than gastric fluid, i.e. their bulk density is less than one. The specific gravity of gastric fluid is approximately 1.004-1.010 g/cm3 according to the "Documenta Geigy" and thus the FDDS remains buoyant in the stomach without affecting the gastric emptying rate for a prolonged period of time. While the system is floating on the gastric contents the drug is released slowly at a desired rate from the system. After the release of the drug the residual system is emptied from the stomach. Some scientists have developed shells of polymers with lower density than that of gastro intestinal fluid to enable them to float. Watanable et al. developed a floating system where they used empty globular shells with a lower density than that of gastrointestinal fluid. This enabled the shells to float on the gastric fluid and to achieve prolonged residence in the stomach. They used polymers such as polystyrene.

I.   **Immediate release system:**

It is the system which releases the drug immediately after administration.

II.   **Extended release system:**

A dosage form that allows at least a twofold reduction in dosage frequency as compared to that drug presented as an immediate release (conventional) dosage form. Allowing a twofold or greater reduction in frequency of administration of a drug in comparison with the frequency required by a conventional dosage form. Various physical and chemical approaches have been successfully applied to produce well-characterized delivery systems that extend drug input into the GI tract within the specifications of the desired release profile. A survey of commercial ER oral solid products indicates that most systems fall into one of three broad categories: matrix, reservoir (or membrane controlled) and osmotic systems. Drug release from these ER delivery systems generally involves one or a combination of the following mechanisms: drug diffusion (through pores of a barrier, through tortuous channels or through a viscous gel layer between polymer chains), system swelling (followed by diffusion and/or erosion and dissolution) or osmotic pressure induced release (drug solution, suspension or wetted mass forced out of the system). Each type of system has its advantages and shortcomings with respect to the performance, applicability, manufacture, control, development time, and cost, etc.

1.4.1.1 Advantages of Extended

1. Avoid patient compliance problem.
2. Employ less total drug
   - Minimize or eliminate local side effects.
   - Minimize or eliminate systemic side effects.
   - Less potential or reduction in activity with chronic use.
   - Minimize drug accumulation with chronic dosing.
3. Improved efficiency in treatment
   - Cure or control of condition more promptly
   - Improved control of condition i.e. less fluctuation in drug level
   - Special effects e.g. sustained release Aspirin provides sufficient drug so that on awakening the arthritic patient has symptomatic relief and another example is sustained release of Salbutamol for early morning relief of asthma by dosing before bedtime.

1.4.1.2 Limitation of Extended Release:

1. Due to formulation defects the extended action dosage form may not release the drug as completely or effectively as expected since the formulation is more complicated than the conventional dosage form.
2. The physician has less flexibility in adjusting dosage regimen. This is fixed by the dosage form design.
3. In case of accidental poisoning it is difficult to administer an antidote.
4. Extended release forms are designed on the basis of average drug biological half-lives. Disease states that alter drug disposition significantly and patient variations are not accommodated.

1.5 Modified Release System

The term modified-release drug product is used to describe products that alter the timing and/or release of the drug substances (fig.1). A modified-release dosage form is defined "as one for which the drug-release characteristics of time course and/or location are chosen to accomplish therapeutic or convenience objectives not offered by conventional dosage forms such as solutions, ointments, or promptly dissolving dosage forms as

24

presently recognized (USP Subcommittee on Biopharmaceutics, 1988).

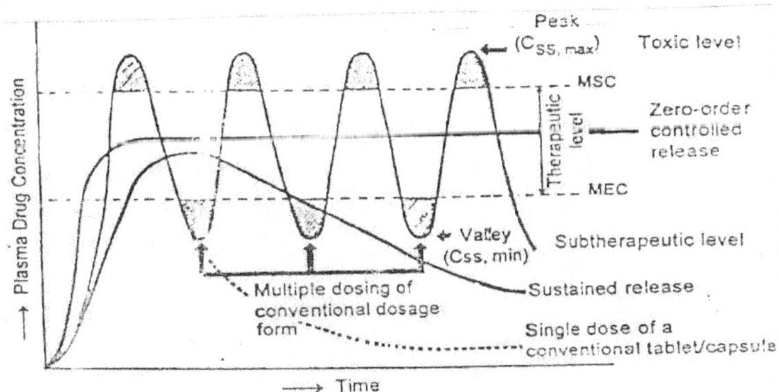

Figure-2 A hypothetical plasma concentration-time profile from conventional multiple dosing and single doses of sustained release and controlled release

Modified release system: (Lordi NG, 2005 and Brahmankar DM, 1995)

1.5.1. Advantages of modified release formulation:

1. Improved patient compliance due to less dosage regimen.

2. Reduction in fluctuation in steady state concentration.

3. Increased safety margin of high potency drugs.

4. Maximum utilization of drug.

5. Reduction in health care cost.

1.5.2 Limitations

1. Decreased systemic availability in certain cases due to incomplete release, insufficient residence time for complete release, site-specific absorption, pH-dependent solubility etc.

2. Poor *In vitro-In vivo* correlation.

3. Possibility of dose dumping.

4. Retrieval of drug is difficult in case of toxicity, poisoning or hypersensitivity reaction.

5. Reduced potential for dosage adjustment of drugs normally administered in varying strengths.

6. Higher cost of formulation.

1.6 Modified Release Dosage Form:

Modified release (MR) drug delivery systems are developed to modulate the apparent absorption Alter the site in order to achieve specific clinical objectives that cannot be attained with conventional dosage forms.

Possible therapeutic benefits of a properly designed MR dosage form include improved efficacy and reduced adverse events, increased convenience and patient compliance, optimized performance, a greater selectivity of activity or new indications.

1.6.1 Types of Modified Release:

1.6.1.1 Sustained Release:

The drug is released slowly at a rate governed by the delivery system. Sustained release systems include any drug delivery, system that achieves slow release of drug over an extended period of time.

A sustained release or a sustained action dosage form is the one which consists of an initial dose part namely loading dose containing sufficient drug to cause a rapid onset of therapeutic response and a sustained release portion namely maintenance dose containing sufficient drug to maintain the initial therapeutic response for the desired number of hours and thus can be maintained provided the release of drug from the dosage form should follow zero-order kinetics i.e. rate of release of the drug is made equal to rate of elimination of the drug.

1.6.1.2 Targeted Release System:

Here the dosage form releases the drug at or near the intended physiologic site of action. Targeted release dosage forms may have either immediate or extended release characteristics.

1.6.1.3 Prolonged Release System

In this the drug product is designed to release the drug slowly and to provide a continuous supply of drug over an extended period. The prolonged action drug products prevent very rapid absorption of drug, which could result in extremely high peak plasma drug concentration.

1.6.1.4 Delayed Release System:

The drug is released at a time other than immediately after administration3 i.e. the site of release is controlled. The dosage form release a discrete portion or portions of drug at a time or times other than promptly after administration although one portion may be released promptly after administration.

A Factors affecting design of modified release drug delivery system

Three aspects that are essential for the development of oral controlled or modified release system are

- Physicochemical properties of the drug and excipients used.

- Relevant GI anatomy and physiology.

- Dosage form characteristics.

(a) Drug properties or physicochemical properties:

Ding X. (2006) mentioned these properties as crystal nature, solubility, intrinsic dissolution, partition coefficient, molecular size, drug stability and protein binding etc. Among all these physicochemical properties, *solubility and membrane permeability* are recognized as fundamental parameters controlling the rate and extent of drug absorption. Biopharmaceutical Drug Classification **(BCS Classification)** proposed by Amidon *et al* defines four categories of therapeutic products based on these two attributes and are shown in Table 1(Shargel L, 2005).

Table 1.

CLASS	SOLUBILITY	PERMEABILITY	IVIVC Expectation
I	High	High	If dissolution rate is slower than gastric emptying rate, otherwise **limited or no correlation**
II	Low	High	If in vitro dissolution rate is similar to in vivo dissolution rate, **IVIVC possible** unless dose is very high
III	High	Low	Permeability is rate determining, **no IVIVC** with dissolution rate
IV	Low	Low	**Limited or no IVIVC**

(b) Aqueous solubility:

The aqueous solubility of a drug influences its dissolution rate, which in turn establishes its concentration in solution and hence the driving force for diffusion across the membrane. Dissolution rate is related to aqueous solubility as shown by the Noyes-Whitney equation (Eq. 1) that under sink conditions is

$$\frac{dc}{dt} = k_D \, A \, C_s \qquad \text{(Eq. 1)}$$

Where dc/dt = Dissolution Rate

k_D = Dissolution Rate Constant

A = Total Surface Area of the Drug Particle

Cs = Aqueous Saturation Solubility of Drug

The dissolution rate is constant only if A remains constant but the important point to be noted is that the initial rate is directly proportional to Cs. Therefore the aqueous solubility of drug can be used as a first approximation of its dissolution rate. Drug with low aqueous solubility have low dissolution rate and usually suffer from oral bioavailability (Ding X, 2006).

(c) pKa

Unionized drugs are absorbed better than ionized ones. In case of weak acids:

$$S_t = S_0 \left(1 + \frac{k_a}{[H^+]} \right) \qquad \text{(Eq. 2)}$$

$$= S_0 \left(1 + 10^{\,pH - pKa} \right) \qquad \text{(Eq. 3)}$$

Where S_t = Total Solubility (both the ionized and unionized form) of weak acid

S_0 = Solubility of unionized form

K_a = Acid Dissociation Constant of conjugated acid.

Equation (2) and (3) show that total solubility of weak acid and weak base with the given pKa can be affected by the pH of the medium. Since weak acid remains unionized in lower pH hence it is absorbed well there, and same is true for weak bases in basic conditions.

eg. Consider the ratio of total solubility of aspirin in the blood and GI fluid as follows:

$$R = \frac{\left(1 + 10^{\,pHb\, -\, pKa}\right)}{\left(1 + 10^{\,pHg\, -\, pKa}\right)} \qquad \text{(Eq. 4)}$$

pHb =   pH of blood (pH 7.4)

pHg =   pH of GI fluid (pH 2)

pKa of aspirin is 3.4

Hence R comes to be $10^{3.8}$ indicating aspirin is readily absorbed within the stomach. The same calculation for intestinal pH (pH 7) yields a ratio close to 1, indicating less driving force for aspirin absorption within small intestine (Ding X., 2006).

Ideally the ratio of an ionizable drug from an extended release system should be programmed in accordance with the variation in pH of the different segments of the absorption forms. Hence delivery system can be formulated as either of the following:

> - Floating formulation
> - Delayed or extended release formulation
> - Targeted drug delivery system.

(d) Partition coefficient

Ding X. (2006) stated that between the times of administration to elimination drug must diffuse through a lipid barrier. This ability of drug is known as membrane permeability.

$$K = \frac{Co}{Cw} \qquad \text{(Eq. 5)}$$

Co = Equilibrium constant of all forms of the drug in

Organic Phase

Cw = Equilibrium constant of all forms of the drug in Aqueous Phase

The relation between permeation and partition coefficient for drug generally is defined by *Hansch Correlation* which describes parabolic relationship between the logarithm of the activity of drug or its ability to be absorbed and logarithm of its partition coefficient. (Fig.2)The value of K at which optimum activity is observed is approx. 1000/1 in n-octanol/water. Drugs with partition coefficient higher or lower than the optimum are poor candidates for ER formulations.

(e) Log *P* **- partition coefficient** (P) describe a chemical's lipophilic or hydrophilic properties and hence also gives good indication about its solubility and absorption.

- *0 and 3 - passive drug absorption.*

- *< 0 - compound is hydrophilic, and hence good solubility but it may*

- *have poor permeability.*

- *> 5 - is highly lipophilic hence favours absorption*

(f) Molecular weight of the drug

Diffusivity is the ability of a drug to diffuse through the membranes is inversely proportional to molecular size. For most polymers it is possible to relate log D empirically to some function of molecular size as follows.

$$\log D = -s_v \log v + k_v \qquad \text{(Eq. 6)}$$

$$= -s_M \log_M + k_m \qquad \text{(Eq. 7)}$$

Where, V = molecular volume

M = molecular weight

sv, sM, kv, km are constants

The upper limit of drug molecular size for passive diffusion is 600 Daltons. For drugs absorbed by pore transport mechanism the molecular size threshold is 150 Daltons for spherical compounds and 400 Daltons for linear compounds. The values of diffusion coefficient corresponding to molecular weight can be seen in following Table 2 (Langer MA, Robinson J. 1990).

Table 2

Molecular weight	Diffusion coefficient (D)
150 – 400 Daltons	10^{-6} to 10^{-9} cm^2/sec. (10^{-8} most common)
> 500 Daltons	Difficult to quantify, that is, less than 10^{-2} cm^2/sec

(g) Drug stability

The stability of the drugs at the site of its release and exposure bio-milieu is one more drug property that can influence the design of oral controlled drug delivery. Drugs that are unstable in gastric pH can be developed as slow release dosage form and drug release can be delayed till the dosage form reaches the intestine. Drugs which undergo gut-wall metabolism and show instability in small intestine are not suitable for oral controlled drug delivery systems (keerman *et al.* 1972). In such cases the drug can be modified chemically to form prodrugs which may possess different physiochemical properties.

(h) Protein binding

Generally the duration of drug action is a function of protein binding. Drug protein binding serves as a depot for the drug molecules. Some drugs such as quaternary ammonium compounds may bind to proteins (mucin) present in the gastrointestinal wall (Leviene, 1961). The drug interaction and the period of binding with mucin like protein also influence the rate and extent of oral absorption.

B. Factors related to polymer

(a) Polymer structure

(Chemical substitution and hydration rate of cellulose)

Methoxy *substitution* is a relatively hydrophobic component and it does not contribute as greatly to the hydrophilic nature of polymer or the rate at which polymer will hydrate. On the other hand the *Hydroxyl Propyl Group* however does contribute greatly to polymer rate of hydration. As a result Methocel *K premium products are fastest to hydrate* because they have lower component of hydrophobic Methoxy substitution and higher amount of hydrophilic Hydroxy Propyl substituent. The range of chemical substitution in Methocel premium product is shown in Table 3

Table 3

Product	% Methoxy Substitution	%Hydroxy-Propyl Substitution	Relative rate of Hydration	USP Type
Methocel K premium	19 – 24	7 – 12	Fastest	HPMC 2208
Methocel E premium	28 – 30	7 – 12	Next Fastest	HPMC 2910
Methocel F premium	27 – 30	4 – 7.5	Slow	HPMC 2906
Methocel A premium	27.5 – 31.5	0	Slowest	HPMC 2208

(b) Polymer level

Hydrophilic matrix containing HPMC absorbs water and swell. The polymer level in outermost hydration layer decreases with time. Bonferoni MC. *et al* (1992) told that the outermost layer of matrix becomes diluted to a point where individual chain detaches from matrix and diffuses into bulk of solution. Polymer chains break away from matrix when the surface concentration passes critical polymer concentration of macro-molecular disentanglement or surface erosion. Wetting is more readily achieved so gel formation is accelerated by varying polymer level (Methocel K4M 10 – 40%), Nellore *et al* (1999) achieved different metoprolol *in vitro* release profile. Sung *et al* (1996) demonstrated that changes in HPMC: Lactose ratio can be used to produce a wide range of drug (Adinazolam Mesylate) release rates. For Methocel 100 Eudragit RSPO matrices, Boza *et al* (1999) showed increase in polymer content resulted in decrease drug release rates due to decrease in total porosity of matrices (initial porosity plus porosity due to dissolution of drug).

(c) Effect of polymer hydration rate

To formulate a successful hydrophilic matrix system one must select a polymer substance that will wet and hydrate to form gelatinous layer fast enough to protect interior of tablets from dissolving and disintegrating during initial wetting and hydration phase. If polymer is too slow to hydrate gastric fluid may penetrate into tablet core dissolve the drug substance and allow the drug substance to diffuse out prematurely. Various grades of commercially available HPMC differ in relative proportion of Hydroxypropyl and Methoxy substitution. Increasing the amount of hydrophilic Hydroxypropyl group leads to faster hydration Methocel *K > Methocel E > Methocel F.* Generally rapid hydrating Methocel K grade is preferred especially for highly water soluble drugs where a rapid rate of hydration is necessary. An inadequate polymer hydration rate may lead to dose dumping due to quick penetration of gastric fluid into tablet.

(d) Molecular weight of polymer

Drug dissolution from the tablet is slower for high molecular weight HPMC polymer. Salomen *et al* (1979) reported that release rate of Potassium Chloride from matrix tablet containing Methocel K100 LV was not different from the release rate from matrix tablet containing K15 M but the higher molecular weight polymer did increase lag time before establishment of quasi-steady state.

(e) Viscosity

Effect of polymer concentration and viscosity can be predicted by Phillipof equation (Eq. 9):

$$v = \{1 + (K + C)\}^8 \qquad \text{(Eq. 9)}$$

Where

v = Viscosity in cps

K = Constant for each individual polymer

C = Concentration expressed as a fraction

In case of HPMC for each grade for fixed polymer level viscosity of selected polymer affects the diffusion and mechanical characteristics of matrix (Cheong LWS *et al.* 1992). By comparing the different Methocel grades Rekhi *et* al (1998) found that higher viscosity gel layer provided a more tortuous and resistant barrier to diffusion which resulted in slower release of drug Metoprolol Hydrochloride.

Snug *et al* (1996) compared different viscosity grades of HPMC (Methocel K100 LV, K15 M and L100 M). The fastest release of Adinazolam Mesylate was achieved for K100 LV formulation. The K4 M formulation exhibited a slightly greater drug release than K15 M and K100 M due to lag of significant difference in release profile between K15 M and K100 M, the authors suggested a limited HPMC viscosity of 15000 cps above which if viscosity was increased the release rate would no longer decrease.

In a study Campos A and Villafuerette R (1997) for low HPMC concentration (10%) formulations the lag time was found to be dependent on viscosity grade. The increasing burst effect produced by higher viscosity grades was attributed to slower swelling with increasing polymer viscosity allowing greater time for dissolution of drug (Metronidazole) before the gel barrier was established. For HPMC concentration of 20% or more the porosity was less important factor in drug release and effect of viscosity was minimized. In case of

 ethyl cellulose the findings were completely different. The lower viscosity grade

resulted in harder tablets and slower release (Katikaneni *et al* 1995)

(f) Effect of polymer particle size

Mitchell K. *et al* (1993) proved that particle size of HPMC polymer can greatly influence polymer performance in hydrophilic matrix. Fraction of HPMC polymer with smaller particle size has more surface area relative to equivalent weight of fraction with larger particle size. Greater surface area provides better polymer water contact thus increasing overall rate at which polymer hydration and gelation occurs. This leads to more effective formation of protective gel barrier which is critical to the performance of hydrophilic matrix tablet.

(g) Polymers used in controlled drug delivery systems

Brannon LP (1997) made a list of materials that can be employed to control the release of drug and other agents. The earliest of these polymers were intended for non-biologicals and were selected because of their desirable physical properties for example:-   Poly urethanes for elasticity

Poly siloxanes or silicons for insulating ability

Poly methyl methacrylate for hydrophilicity and strength

Poly ethylene for toughness

Poly vinyl pyrrolidine for suspension capabilities

It must have an appropriate structure with minimal undesired character of aging and should be readily processable. Some of these which are currently being used or studied for control drug delivery include

Poly 2-hydroxyethyl methacrylate

Poly N-vinyl pyrrolidone

Poly methyl methacrylate

Poly acryl acid

Poly vinyl alcohol

Poly acrylamide

Poly ethylene covinyl acetate

Poly ethylene glycol

Poly methacrylic acid

However in recent years additional polymers designed for medical application have entered in the area of controlled release formulations. Many of these materials are designed to get degraded within the body itself some of those are:

Poly lactides (PLA)

Poly glycolides (PGA)

Poly lactide-co-glycolides (PLGA)

Poly anhydrides

The polymers used in controlled release formulations can also be categorized into two types swellable and non-swellable. Swellable polymers are water insoluble and also called *hydro-gels*. They include HPMC While non-swellable are water soluble and called *hydrophilic matrices*. They include Eudragit (Ranga Rao KV. 1998).

C. Other technological variables

(a) Effect of filler

Zhang YW *et al* (2000) showed that addition of water soluble filler can actually increase viscosity of gel because it affects the amount of water available to help the polymer to thicken by adding insoluble material to hydrophilic matrix a slower release rate can be achieved that might not be expected without filler. Rekhi *et al* 1998 studied the effect of filler (57% of tablet weight) on Metoprolol formulation at 20% Methocel K4 M level.

(b) Surfactants

Feely and Devis (1988) characterized the ability of charged ionic surfactants to retard the releases of oppositely charged drugs for HPMC tablets (Chlorpheniramine Maleate and Sodium Alkyl Sulphates, Sodium Salicylate, and Potassium Phenoxy Methyl Penicillin) from HPMC matrix (85% nonionic polymers at 15% of tablet weight) did not significantly alter the release rates. Sodium CMC (50% replacement of HPMC) reduced the Chlorpheniramine Maleate release in pH 7 buffer (near zero order release) but not in acidic medium. This was explained by complexation of drug with cationic polymer which was not possible below pH 3 when sodium CMC was in its unionized insoluble form. As a result of the complexation the gel erosion became prominent release mechanism instead of diffusion. No interaction occurred between sodium Salicylate and sodium CMC (both are anionic).

In the presence of diethyl amino dextran, Sodium Salicylate release was slower at pH 7 but did not alter at pH 1 (when the drug was in its unionized form). Overall the effect of ionic polymers incorporated in HPMC matrices on the release of oppositely charged drugs was small compared to ion exchange resins. Takka *et al* (2001) studied the effect of addition of anionic polymers (Eudragit S, Eudragit L100 and Sodium CMC) on release of weakly basic drugs.

D. Process variables

(a) Compression Force

It has been reported by Velasco *et al* (1999) that for HPMC tablet that although the compression force has significant effect on tablet hardness its effect on drug release from HPMC tablet was minimal. It could be assumed that the variation in compression force should be closely related to change in the porosity of tablets. However as the porosity of hydration matrix is independent of the initial porosity the compression force seems to have little influence on drug release. The influence of compression force could only be observed in lag time. Rekhi *et al* (1999) reported similar findings i.e. changes in compression force or crushing strength appeared to have minimal effect on drug release from HPMC matrix tablet once a critical hardness is achieved. Increased dissolution was only observed when tablets were too soft and it was attributed to the lack of powder compaction or consolidation (3 KP).

(b) Tablet shape

Rekhi *et al* (1999) & Siepnamm J. *et al* (2000) showed that size and shape of tablet for the matrix system undergoing diffusion and erosion might affect the drug dissolution rate. Modification of surface area for Metoprolol Tartarate tablets formulated with Methocel K100 LV from standard concave shape (0.568 sq in) to caplet shape (0.747 sq in) showed an approximately 20 – 30% increase in dissolution at each time point. Furthermore they recommended that for maximum maintenance of controlled release characteristics tablet matrices should be as near spherical as possible to produce minimal release rate.

1.7 Release of drug from formulation

1.7.1 Release rate

Ding X (2006) reported that the conventional dosage forms can be considered to release their active ingredients into an absorption pool immediately. This is illustrated by the following simple kinetic scheme.

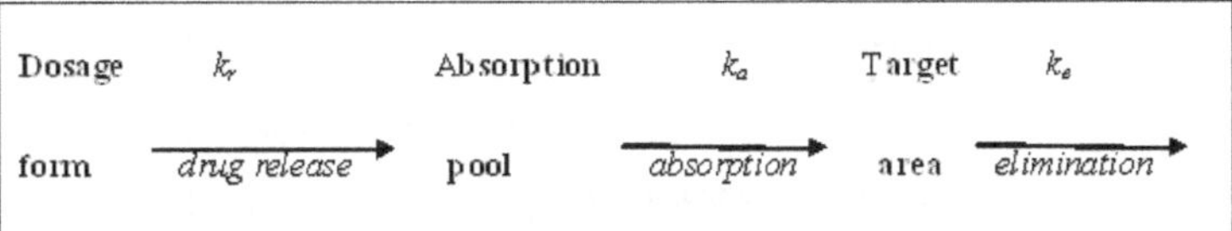

The absorption pool represents a solution of the drug at the site of absorption and the term k_r, k_a, k_e are first order rate constants for drug release absorption and overall elimination respectively. Immediate release form implies that $k_r >>> k_a$ or alternatively the absorption of drug across a biological membrane such as the intestinal epithelium is the rate limiting step in delivery of the drug to its target area. For non-immediate release dosage forms $k_r <<< k_a$, i.e. release of drug from dosage form is the rate limiting step. This causes above kinetic scheme to reduce.

1.7.2 Release order

Jantzen GM. (2005) told that the release of the drug from any matrix tablet can follow either of the two orders

- Zero order release rate

- First order release rate

1.7.3 Design and fabrication of controlled release products

Extensive reviews are available on ways to design a sustained release dosage form.

1.7.3.1 Diffusion-controlled system

According to Baker R. (1987) in diffusion-controlled system a substance is released from a device by permeation from its interior to the surrounding medium. The rate of diffusion of the agent into the system governs its rate of release. It can be further of following types:

1.7.3.2 Reservoir devices

Baker R., (1987) has mentioned this system as the simplest diffusion controlled system. An inert membrane encloses the agent to be released the agent diffuses through the membrane at a finite controllable rate. This type of system has the advantage of providing a constant rate of release over a substantial portion of their lifetime.

1.7.3.3 Monolithic devices

In monolithic devices the material to be released is dispersed uniformly throughout the rate controlling polymer medium. According to Baker R (1987) the release profile is then determined by the loading of dispersed agent the nature of the components and the geometry of the device.

These systems can be either *monolithic solution type* (where the active agent due to its free solubility in polymer medium is dissolved in polymer medium) or *monolithic dispersion type* (due to more limited solubility of active agent in polymer medium only a portion of the agent is dissolved in the polymer medium and the remainder is dispersed as small particles throughout the polymer).

1.7.3.4 Swelling-controlled device

The reservoir and monolithic systems both involve the rate of diffusion of agent through a rate-limiting membrane or matrix. It is assumed that these membranes do not change during the release process. This is not always the case and a class of devices exists in which absorption of solvent (water) from the outside environment changes the rate controlling membrane and thus the agent release kinetics. This system by Baker R (1987) is called as swelling-controlled system. For example consider a polymer hydrogel containing disperse water-soluble agent. Initially the diffusion coefficient of agent in the dehydrated hydrogel is very low but increases significantly as the gel imbibes water. Agent release from the device is thus a function of the rate of uptake of water from surrounding media and the rate of drug diffusion.

1.8 Types of oral controlled release systems: (Vyas SP, 2002)

It can be of following types

- Matrix tablets
- Plastic Matrices
- Ion-Exchange Resin Tablets
- Film-Coated Tablets
- Enteric-Coated and Delayed Release Tablets
- Floating Tablets
- Mucoadhesive Tablets
- Osmotic Tablets

- Repeat-Action Tablets
- Floating Capsules
- Microgranules and Spheroids
- Beads
- Pellets
- Microcapsule and Microspheres

1.9. Release mode from matrix release tablet

This swelling controlled system shows two types of diffusion patterns.

1.9.1. Simple Fickian diffusion

Subrahmanyam CVS (2005) told that diffusion of solvent into the device follows Fick's law (Eq. 11) which states that the flux (the rate of mass transfer across a unit surface area of barrier) is directly proportional to the concentration gradient.

$$J = -D \frac{dC}{dx} \qquad \text{(Eq. 11)}$$

Where,

J = permeation flux (g/cm^2 sec)

dC/dx = concentration gradient in the membrane.

D = diffusion coefficient.

The minus sign reflects the fact that the direction of flow is down the gradient in conc. As per Baker R (1987) the rate of absorption of solvent during the first 60% of the total absorption ion is given by following equation:

$$\frac{M_{s(t)}}{M_{s(0)}} = 4\left(\frac{Dt}{\pi l^2}\right)^{1/2} \qquad \text{(Eq. 12)}$$

Where, $M_{s(0)}$ = total mass of the solvent sorbed by the device when it is equilibrated.

$M_{s(t)}$ = total mass of the solvent sorbed by the device at time t.

l = thickness of the device.

D = diffusion coefficient.

The solvent concentration profiles formed in are shown in graph below for such a device (Fig.3) predicting the effect of the rate of water sorption on the rate of release of dispersed agent is difficult. The agent release rate is governed by the dependence of the diffusion coefficient of the particular agent on polymer water content. In spite of these complexities this type of release system is quite widely used in oral tablet formulations. The principle component of the tablet is usually a dry hydrophilic matrix in which drug is dispersed. After ingestion the tablet swells and slowly releases the drug

1.9.2 Non-Fickian case II diffusion

A second and more predictable type of swelling-controlled system utilizes "Non-Fickian Case II" type diffusion. This terminology was first used by Alfery to describe diffusion in which the diffusion coefficient depends strongly on both concentration and time. In this type the rate of solvent uptake into a polymer is largely determined by the rate of swelling and relaxation of the polymer chains (Baker R., 1987).Arno EA et al (2002) explained that since hydrophilic polymers like Carbopol and HPMC can easily take in water and can swell because of structural relaxation it is possible to modulate the drug release which depends on the interaction between water polymer and drug. As a result an outer gel layer is formed producing physical changes in the matrix that can be observed through the behavior of different fronts as the process develops. These fronts have been identified (Fig.3) as;

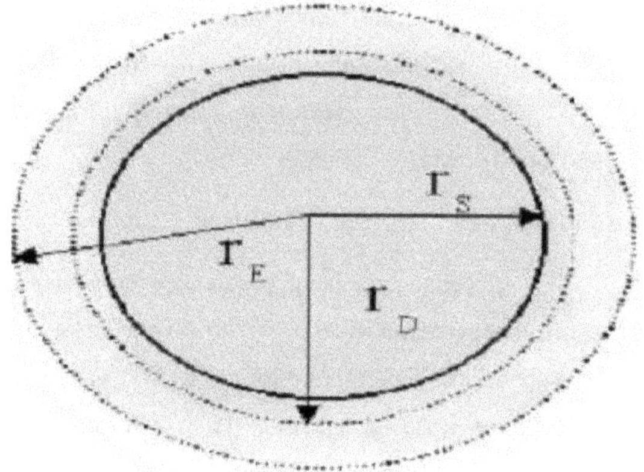

Figure- 3 Different fronts formed during swelling diffusion.

1.9.3. Dissolution specification for controlled release systems:

For ER formulation FIP guidelines demand at least three specification point of drug release: (Sievert B, Sielwert M. 2000)

- ❖ After 1-2 hr 20-30% to provide assurance against premature drug release.
- ❖ Around 50% to define dissolution pattern.

- ❖ At least 80% to ensure almost quantitative release.

1.9.4 Purpose of establishing dissolution specifications-

- ❖ To ensure batch-to-batch consistency within range.

- ❖ To guarantee acceptable performance *in- vivo.*

- ❖ To distinguish between good and bad batches.

1.9.5. Mathematical analysis of drug release

Quantitative interpretation of the values obtained in dissolution assays is easier by using mathematical equation which describes the release profile as a function of some parameter related with pharmaceutical dosage forms. Some of the most relevant and more commonly used mathematical models describing the dissolution curves are as follows: (Higuchi T. 1963)

Zero order: $\qquad Q_t = Q_0 + K_0 t$ $\qquad$ (Eq. 14)

Hixon-Crowell: $Q_0^{1/3} - Q_t^{1/3} = K_s t$ $\qquad$ (Eq. 15)

Higuchi: $\qquad Q_t = K_n t$ $\qquad$ (Eq. 16)

Korsemeyer-Peppas: $Q_t / Q_0 = K_k t^n$ $\qquad$ (Eq. 17)

The Higuchi and Zero Order models (Eq. 14) represent two limit cases in transport and drug release phenomenon and the Korsemeyer-Peppas model (Eq. 17) is a decision parameter between these two models. While Higuchi model (Eq. 16) has larger application in polymeric systems the Zero Order Model becomes ideal to describe coated dosage forms or membrane controlled forms. One common method uses the coefficient of determination r^2 to assess the "fit" of model equation. Besides the coefficient of determination r^2 the correlation coefficient (r) the sum square of residues (SSR), the mean square error (MSE) and the F-ratio probability are also used to test the applicability of the release models.

Generally after the application of the melt the granules are cooled rapidly which sometimes results in cracks in the coating because of contraction of the coating material. These cracks can further increase during compression of granules into tablets due to higher compression forces. This non-uniformity of coating and cracks formed during cooling and compression can lead to variation in drug release from tablet to tablet/batch to batch and thus can affect the desired blood levels or complete failure of the system leading to dose dumping.

Chapter-2

Drug Profile

2.1 Drug Name –Cephalexin

These are a group of semisynthic antibiotics derived from 'Cephalosporin-c' obtained from a fungus cephalosporium.These are chemically related to penicillins;the nucleus consists of a beta-lactam ring to dihydrothizine ring (7-aminocephalosporanic acid).By addition of different side chain at position 7 of beta-lactam ring and position 3 of dihydrothizine ring (affecting pharmacokinetics),alarge number of semisynthetic compounds have been produced.Cephalexin is an orally active, first generation cephalosporin antibiotic,similar in spectrum to cephalothin but less active against penicillinase producing staphylococci and against H.influenzae.It is little bound to plasma proteins,attains high concentration in bile and is excreted unchanged in urine;t1\2 ~60 min.It is effective against gram-positive organism, while having limited gram-negative coverage. Cephalexin is used in the treatment of pharyngitis, tonsillitis, urinary tract infection and uncomplicated skin infection.

2.2 Chemical Structure:

2.3 Chemical Name: (7R)-3-Methyl-7-(alpha-D-*phenylglycylamino*)-3-cephem-4-Carboxylic acid monohydrate

2.4 Molecular Formula: $C_{16} H_{17} N_3 O_4 S$

2.5 Solubility:

Solvent Cephalexin monohydrate/ml	Mg.
Water	14.5
Methanol	4.4
n-Octanol	0.03
Chloroform	<0.01

Ether	<0.01

2.6 Mechanism of action:

Cephalexin is a bactericidal antibiotic that inhibits bacterial cell wall synthesis by binding to one or more penicillin binding proteins of actively dividing cells. It is also proposed that Cephalosporin decrease the availability of an inhibitor to murein hydrolase (autolysin), an enzyme involved in cell division.

2.7 Physical properties: 1.16 g of cephalexin hydrochloride monograph substance is approximately equivalent to 1 g of anhydrous cephalexin.

2.8 Appearance: White to off-white, crystalline powder.

2.9 Odor: Characteristic

2.10 pH: 5% aqueous suspension is between 4.0-5.5

1% aqueous solution is between 1.5-4.0

2.11 Molecular Weight: 347.393

2.12 pKa: 4.2

2.13 Storage And Stability:

Tablets, Capsules, Powder for oral suspension store in tight container at room temperature 15-30^{0}c Reconstituted oral suspension stable for 2 weeks.

2.14 Pharmacokinetics:

Route	:	Oral
Bioavailability	:	90%
Half Life	:	.9hrs
Metabolism	:	90% unchanged
Excretion	:	Renal

2.15 Therapeutics:

Cephalexin is a first-generation cephalosporin that displays activity against *Streptococcal* and *Staphylococcal* species. It has limited gram-negative activity against some strains of *Escherichia coli*, *Klebsiella pneumonia*, and *Proteus mirabilis*.

2.16 Dosage:

250 mg every 6 hrs & can be administered as 500 mg every 12hrs.

2.17 Contraindications:

Cephalexin is contraindicated in patients with a history of allergic reactions to cephalosporin antibiotics. Cephalexin should be avoided in those with anaphylactic reactions to penicillin's and should be used with caution in patients with delayed hypersensitivity reactions such as rash, fever, or eosinophilia.

2.18 Brand Name's: *Keflex, Sporidex, Nufex.*

2.19 Formulation Available:

2.19.1 Oral: Tablets, Capsules, and powder for reconstitution

2.19.2 Injectable: Sodium salt (Seprox$^®$ injection Glaxovet) for IM & SC use

Excipient Profile

Magnesium stearate

Magnesium stearate is a fine, white, precipitated or milled, impalpable powder of low bulk density, having a faint odor of Stearic acid and a characteristic taste. The powder is greasy to touch and readily adheres to the skin.

Empirical formula: $C_{36}H_{70}MgO_4$

Molecular weight: 591.34

Structural formula: $[CH_3\,(CH_2)_{16}COO]_2Mg$

Functional category: Tablet and capsule lubricant.

Applications in this formulation:

It is primarily used as a lubricant at concentrations between 0.25-5.0 percent. Magnesium stearate is used as lubricant for tableting for example 1% magnesium stearate or 1% sodium stearyl fumarate. Though Maltodextrin appears to have no adverse effect on the rate of dissolution of tablet, magnesium stearate 0.5-1.0% may be used as a lubricant (Kibbe AH 2000).

Purpose.

The objective of this study was to determine the effects of magnesium stearate (lubricant) concentration on the compression properties of coprocessed excipients. The Lubricant sensitivity ratio (LSR) was determined. To obtain evidence on the lubricant film formation around excipient particles during the mixing process.

Methods.

Physical and reological evaluations were made for all coprocessed excipients including flow rate (flowability) and repose angle. Physical mixtures of excipient and magnesium stearate at 0, 0.5, and 1.0% were preparated on a V-shape mixer operating at 25 rpm. Secondary electron microscopy was used to study the morphology and texture of original particles(withoutlubricant), and the lubricant film formation on the base carrier material. Tableting was carried out on a hydraulic Press (Carver), using 13 mm diameter die and flat faced punches, at applied pressures of 88.3, 132.4, 176.6, 264.8, and 353.1 MPa. Tablet weight was 600 mg. Tablet crushing strength (kp) was determined, and the LSR calculated.

Results.

The addition of 0.5% of magnesium stearate caused a significative decreasing on compactability for all coprocessed excipients. The effect of higher lubricant concentrations was less evident. At 88.3 Mpa and 0.5% magnesium stearate, the LSR expressed as percentage was 25.3%, 18.3%, 12.2%, and 9.3% for StarLac, Ludipress, Cellactose 80 and MicroceLac 100 respectively. At 88.3 Mpa and 1.0% magnesium stearate, the LSR expressed as percentage was 36.2%, 24.9%, 14%, and 9.5% for StarLac, Ludipress, Cellactose 80 and MicroceLac 100 respectively. The highest sensitivity was showed by StarLac. In contrast, MicroceLac showed the lower LSR. As compaction pressure increased the LSR decreased. Lubricant films on host particles were detected by SEM. Preferential deposition zones were observed. Preferential deposition zones were observed.

Conclusion.

Magnesium stearate forms an adsorbed lubricant film around excipient particles. This physical barrier decreased the crushing strength of all tablets. The effect depends on the coprocessed excipient used. StarLac resulted more sensitive and MicroceLa less sensitive to lubricant. Preferential deposition zones were observed.

Lactose

Lactose. Freely but slowly soluble in water practically insoluble in ethanol (95 per cent). Lactose Monohydrate Milk Sugar

Empirical formula: $C_{12}H_{22}O_{11}, H_2O$

Structural formula:

Mol.Wt. :   360.3

Lactose is O-β-D-galactopyranosyl-(1 → 4)-α – Dglucopyranose monohydrate.

Polymer Used

Hydroxypropyl methylcellulose

Hydroxypropyl methylcellulose is an odorless and tasteless, white or creamy-white colored fibrous or granular powder. The PhEur describes Hydroxypropyl methylcellulose as a partly O-methylated and O-(2-hydroxypropylated) cellulose. It is available in several grades which vary in viscosity and extent of substitution. Grades may be distinguished by appending a number indicative of the apparent viscosity in mPa s of a 2% w/w aqueous solution at 20 °C.

Molecular weight: approximately 10,000-1 5, 00,000.

Structural formula:

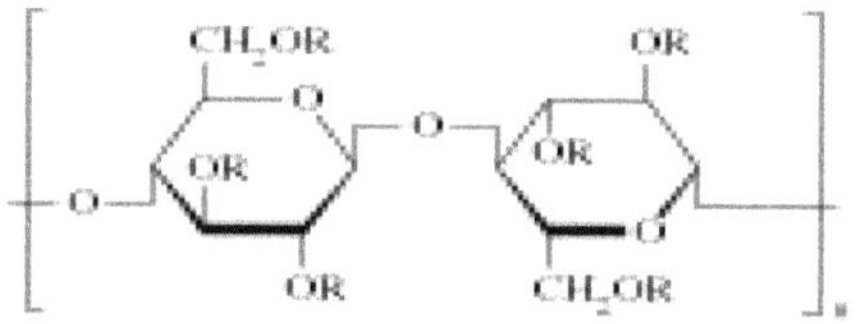

Where,

$$R = H, CH_3, \text{ or } [CH_3CH(OH)CH_2]$$

Functional category:

Rate-controlling polymer for sustained release, tablet binder, Coating agent, film-former, stabilizing agent, suspending agent, viscosity-increasing agent.

Applications in this formulation:

It is primarily used as a tablet binder and as an extended-release (Dahl TC. 1990) tablet matrix in a concentration of 2-5% w/w to retard the release of drugs from matrix at levels 10-80% w/w.

Eudragit

1. Commercial form

Solid substance obtained from EUDRAGIT L 30 D-55.

The product contains 0.7% Sodium Laurilsulfate Ph.Eur./NF and 2.3% Polysorbate -80 Ph. Eur. / NF on solid substance, as emulsifiers. Eudragit L 100 55 is described in the monographs quoted above.

2. Chemical structure

Eudragit L 100-55 contains an anionic copolymer based on methacrylic acid and ethyl acrylate.

The ratio of the free carboxyl groups to the ester groups is approx. 1:1. The average molecular weight is approx. 250,000.

3. CharactersSS

Description

White powder with a faint characteristic odour.

Solubility

1 g of Eudragit L 100-55 dissolves in 7 g methanol, ethanol, isopropyl alcohol and acetone, as well as in 1 N sodium hydroxide to give clear to slightly cloudy solutions. Eudragit L 100-55 is practically insoluble in ethyl acetate, methylene chloride, petroleum ether and water.

4. Tests

Test solution

A 12.5 % solution of the dry substance in isopropyl alcohol/water is used for the Test solution: a quantity of Eudragit L 100-55 corresponding to 12.5 g dry substance is dissolved in a mixture of 84.9 g isopropyl alcohol and 2.6 g water.

Particle size

At least 95 % less than 0.25 mm.

Chapter-3

Preformulation Studies

Preformulation activities range from supporting identification of new active agents to characterize physical properties necessary for the design of dosage forms. Critical information provided during the preformulation can enhance the rapid and successful introduction of new therapeutic entities for humans. Hence, preformulation studies are essential to characterize drugs for proper designing of drug delivery system. The preformulation studies, which were performed in this project include- identification of drugs (physical appearance, determination of melting point, IR spectra and UV absorption maxima), quantitative solubility studies, and estimation of drug.

3.1 Tests for identification of Cephalexin

3.1.1 Physical appearance

White to off-white crystalline powder.

3.1.2 Melting point

The melting point of the drug was determined using melting point apparatus (Tempo, India) and found to be sharp at 336.8°C.

3.1.3 Solubility studies

Solubility may be defined as the spontaneous interaction of two or more substances to form a homogenous dispersion (Sethi, 1985). The solubility of drug was studied in various solvents. The solubility of drug is an important physicochemical property because it affects the bioavailability, drug release into the dissolution medium, and consequently, the therapeutic efficacy of the pharmaceutical product.

For quantitative solubility studies, unknown amount of drug (10 mg) was suspended in a series of different solvents and shaken for 24 hr using Wrist Action

Shaker (York, India). The solubility of Cephalexin in different solvents is recorded in Table 3.1.

Table 3.1: Solubility of Cephalexin in different solvents

S. No.	Solvent	Solubility
1	Water	++
2	0.1N NAOH	− −
3	Dimethyl formamide	+++
4	PBS (pH 5.6)	+
5	PBS (pH 7.4)	-
6	Ethanol	+
7	Methanol	− −
8	Chloroform	− −
9	Acetone	−
10	DCM	− −

11	Tetrahydrofuran	+++

+++, Freely soluble (< 1 part); ++, Soluble (1-10 parts); +, sparingly soluble (10-30 parts); -, practically insoluble (>10,000 parts)

3.1.4 Partition coefficient

Partition coefficient is a measure of drug lipophilicity that gives an indication about its ability to cross the biomembranes. It can be defined as the ratio of unionized drug distributed between the organic and aqueous phase at equilibrium.

$$Po/w = [C_{org}/C_{aq}] \text{ equilibrium}$$

Drugs having values of P much greater than 1 are classified as lipophilic, whereas those with partition coefficient much less than 1 are indicative of a hydrophilic drug.

3.1.4.1 Partition coefficient of drug in n-Octanol: Distilled water

The partition coefficient of drug was determined in n-octanol: PBS (pH 7.4) and n-octanol: Distilled water by flask shaking method (BPC, 1979). Accurately weighted 10 mg of drug was transferred into glass stoppered test tubes containing 10 ml each n-octanol and respective aqueous phase (PBS 5.6/distilled water). The test tubes were placed on a wrist action shaker (York, India) for 24 hrs. Both phases were separated using separating funnel and the aqueous phase was analyzed for the amount of drug after suitable dilution. The log of ratio of drug concentration in n-octanol:water is shown in the table3.2.

Table 3.2: Partition coefficient of Cephalexin in different systems

S. No.	System	Partition coefficient (logP)
1	n-octanol:distilled water	6.24±.0264
2	n-octanol:PBS (pH 5.6)	6.56±0.018

(n=3)

3.1.4.2 Partition coefficient of drug in Skin: PBS (pH 5.6)

Skin:PBS pH 5.6 partition coefficient was determined using the method reported by Valia, *et al.*, 1985 and Tojo *et al.,* (1987). A 100 mg piece of excised rat skin was weighted accurately and kept in a glass stoppered test tube containing 10 ml mixture of PBS (pH 5.6) and PEG 400 in 80:20 ratio. The accurately weighted (10 mg) drug was added to this system. Mixture was equilibrated for 24 hr at 37+1°C. The solution was filtered and the drug concentration was determined spectrophotometrically at λmax 268 nm. The log of ratio of drug concentration in skin: PBS (7.4) is shown in the table 3.2.

3.1.5 Determination of absorption maxima (λmax)/wavelength maxima

Accurately weighed 10 mg of Cephalexin was dissolved in 2 ml dimethylformamide (DMF) then the volume was made upto 100 mL with methano in a 100 mL volumetric flask. Then, 1 mL of this stock solution was pipetted into a 10 mL volumetric flask and volume made up with methanol:water(20:1). The resulting solution was then scanned between 260-280 nm using UV-visible spectrophotometer (Shimadzu 1601 UV, Japan). The λmax was found to be 268 nm.

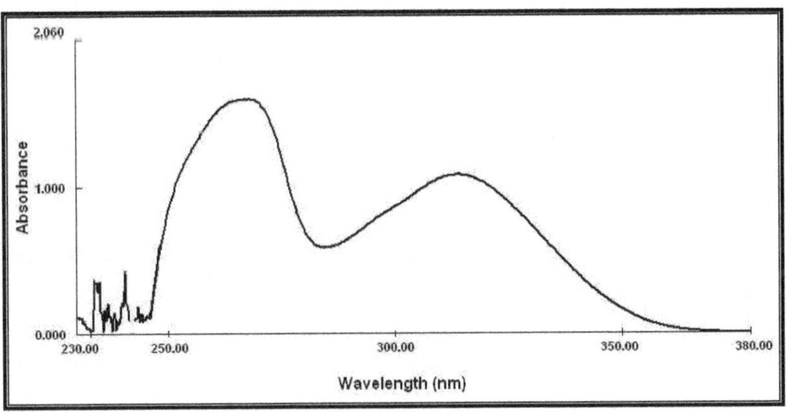

Figure 3.1 UV spectrum of cephalexin in methanol

3.1.6 Infra Red Spectrum

IR spectrum of any compound or drug gives information about the groups present in that particular compound. IR spectrum of the drug sample was obtained using IR spectrophotometer (FTIR Perkin Elmer, Pyrogon-1000, USA fig-3.2) and the obtained peaks were interpreted for presence of different functional groups.

Table- 3.3 show few Important band frequencies in FTIR spectrum of Cephalexin.

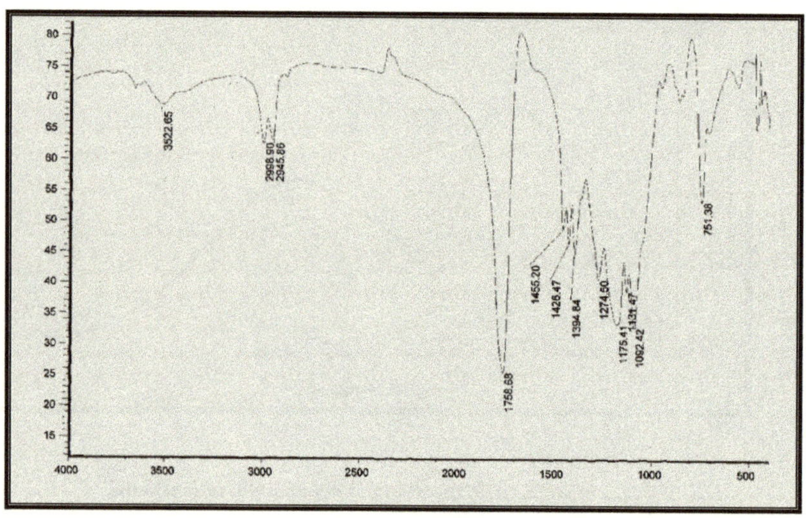

Figure 3.2: FTIR spectrum of cephalexin

Table 3.3: Important band frequencies in FTIR spectrum of Cephalexin

Observed Band Frequency cm^{-1}	Vibration Mode	Tentative Assignments
3522	O-H Stretching	Presence of carboxyl group
2998.90	C-H Stretching	Presence of Aromatic Stretching Group
2945.66	C-H Stretching	Presence of cycloalkane ring (adamantyl group) and methyl guoup.
1758.68	C=O Stretching	Presence of carbonyl group of carboxylic acid
1455.20	C=C Stretching	Presence of Ring Skeleton
1426	O-H Bending	Presence of carboxylic group
1394.84	C-H Bending	Presence of methyl group and aliphatic ring
1274	C-O stretching	Presence of carboxylic group
1175.41,113.47	C-C stretching	Presence of cycloalkanes
1092.42	C-C stretching	Presence of cycloalkanes

751.38	Out of plane C-H bending	Presence of olefinic group in aromatic ring

3.2 Estimation of drug

3.2.1 Standard curve of Cephalexin

Accurately weighted 10 mg drug was taken in a 100 ml volumetric flask and 2 ml DMF was added to it. Then methanol was added to above solution make the volume to 100 ml and a stock solution of 100 $\mu g/ml$ was prepared. From this stock 0.2, 0.4........ 2.0 ml were withdrawn in a series of 10 ml volumetric flasks and diluted to 10.0 ml with methanol. This gave solution in a final concentration range of 2-20 $\mu g/ml$. The absorbance of each solution was determined at λ_{max} 268 nm using UV spectrophotometer and observation is recorded in table 3.4

Table 3.4: Standard curve of Cephalexin in methanol at λmax268nm.

S.No	Conc. μg/mL	Abstorbance at λ =268nm	Regressed values	Equation of line
1	2	0.1647	0.1677	
2	4	0.313	0.3253	
3	6	0.4871	0.4829	
4	8	0.6536	0.6405	
5	10	0.7948	0.7981	Y=.0788X+.0101
6	12	0.9675	0.9557	R2= 0.9995
7	14	1.1096	1.1133	
8	16	1.2843	1.2709	
9	18	1.4116	1.4285	
10	20	1.5867	1.5861	

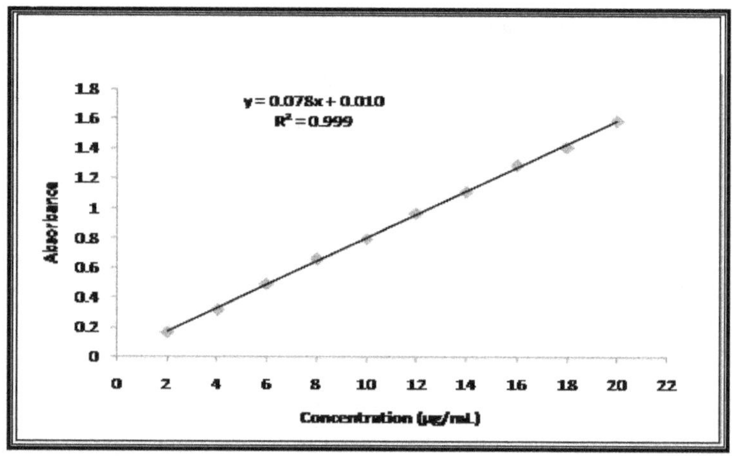

Figure 3.3 calibration curve of cephalexin methanol

Accurately weighted 10 mg drug was taken in a 100 ml volumetric flask and 2 ml DMF was added to it. Then mixture of (ratio4:1) methanol:PBS (pH5.6) was added to above solution to make the volume to 100 ml and a stock solution of 100 µg/ml was prepared. From this stock 0.2, 0.4…….. 2.0 ml were withdrawn in a series of 10 ml volumetric flasks and diluted to 10.0 ml with (ratio4:1) methanol:PBS(pH5.6). This gave solution in a final concentration range of 2-20 µg/ml. The resulting solutions were filtered through whatman filter paper no.1 and the absorbance of each solution was determined at λ_{max} 268 nm using UV spectrophotometer and observation is recorded in Table 3.5.

Table 3.5: Standard curve of Cephalexin in PBS (pH5.6):methanol at λmax268nm.

S.No	Concentration in μg/mL	Absorbance at λ =268 nm	Regressed values	Equation of line
1	2	0.182	0.137	
2	4	0.346	0.321	
3	6	0.497	0.505	
4	8	0.686	0.689	
5	10	0.824	0.873	Y=.092X-0.047
6	12	0.982	1.057	R^2= 0.995
7	14	1.235	1.241	
8	16	1.467	1.425	
9	18	1.625	1.609	
10	20	1.834	1.793	

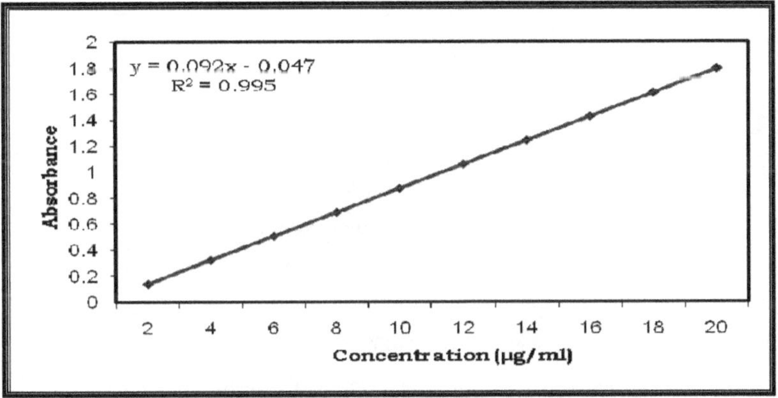

Figure 3.4 Linearly regressed standard curve of
***Cephalexin* in methanol: PBS (pH 5.6)**

3.3 Validation of Cephalexin

(1) *Linearity*

A stock solution of Cephalexin (1000 ng/µL) was prepared in Water. Different volumes of stock solution, 0.5, 0.8, 1, 1.2, 1.5 µL were spotted on TLC plate to obtain concentration of 500, 800, 1000, 1200, 1500 ng per spot of Cephalexin, respectively. The data of peak area v/s drug amount were treated by linear least-square regression analysis.

(2) Analysis of the marketed formulation

To determine the content of Cephalexin in tablets (label claim: 125 mg per tablet). Twenty tablets were powdered and powder equivalent to 25 mg was weighed and transfered to a 25 ml volumetric flask containing about 20 ml water, the solution was filtered through whatman filter paper and finally volume was made upto 25 ml to get the stock solution of (1000 ng/µL) Appropriate volume of solution was applied on TLC plate followed by development and scanning.

(3) Forced degradation Studies

A stock solution containing 25 mg Cephalexin in 25 ml distilled water was prepared. This solution was used for forced degradation.

a. Degradation under acid catalysed hydrolytic condition

To 2.5 ml stock solution, 2.5 ml of 0.1 N HCl was added. The volume was made upto 25 ml with distilled water. The mixture was refluxed at 80 o C for one hour.

Appropriate volume of resultant solution (1000 ng per spot) was applied on TLC plate and densitograms were developed.

b. Degradation under alkali catalysed hydrolytic condition

To 2.5 ml stock solution, 2.5 ml of 0.01 N NaOH was added. The volume was made upto 25 ml with distilled water. This mixture was kept at room temperature for half hour. Appropriate volume of resultant solution (1000 ng per spot) was applied on TLC plate and densitograms were developed.

c. Degradation under neutral hydrolytic condition

To 2.5 ml stock solution, distilled water was added. The volume was made upto 25 ml. The mixture was refluxed for 15 min at 80 0 C. Appropriate volume of resultant solution (1000 ng per spot) was applied on TLC plate and densitograms were developed.

d. Degradation under oxidative condition

To 2.5 ml stock solution, 2.5 ml of 30 % H2O2 was added. The volume was made upto 25 ml with distilled water. The mixture was kept at room temperature for 3 days. Appropriate volume of resultant solution (1000 ng per spot) was applied on TLC plate and densitograms were developed.

3.4 Stress degradation of Formulation

Cephalexin tablets, each containing 125 mg Cephalexin were purchased from local market, The tablets were weighed, crushed and sample powder was exposed to stress condition as mentioned under study for bulk drugs. Then the sample was filtered & appropriate volume was spotted on to TLC plate. Fig-3.5

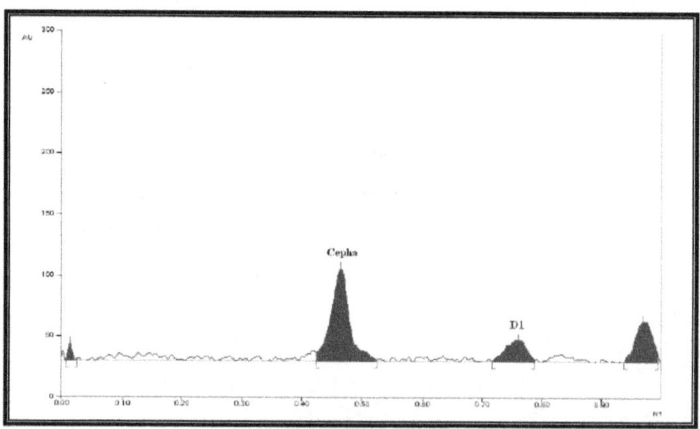

Fig. 3.5 Densitogram of Cephalexin and its degradation products after acid catalysed hydrolysis

3.5. Compatibility Study

Drug compatibility with phosphatidyl choline (PC), and lipid tristearin(GTS) was also checked. Solution of adapalene ($10\mu g$) was prepared in PBS (pH 5.6). Accurately weighed lipid 10 mg of lipid transferred separately into 10 mL volumetric flasks containing drug solution. Absorbance was measured for each solution using Cintra-10 UV Spectrophotometer against respective blank solution. The absorbance values are presented in table 3.6

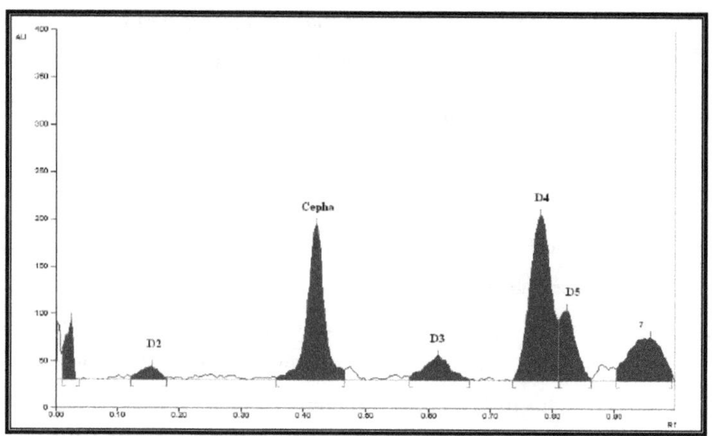

Fig. 3.6 Densitogram of Cephalexin and its degradation products after base catalysed hydrolysis.

Table 3.6 compatibility study of Cephalexin with formulation ingredients

S.No.	Composition	Absorption maxima (λmax in nm)	Absorbance
1.	**Cephalexin**	268	0.7126
2.	**Cephalexin + HPMC**	268	0.6987
3.	**Cephalexin +Lactose**	268	0.7264

3.6. Results and Discussion

Identification studies showed that the drug supplied by Ranbaxy Lab. Ltd. Dewas M.P., matches with the standards as prescribed in Europian pharmacopoeia 2006. The drug supplied was white or almost white, crystalline powder. The IR spectrum of Cephalexin shows different band frequencies which are concordant with functional group present in it.

Solubility profile of the drug in different solvents at room temperature indicates that the drug was soluble in dimethylformamide, tetrahydrofuran, Spingly soluble in water, PBS (pH7.4), methanol, chloroform, acetnone,0.1NaoH and sparingly soluble in PBS (pH5.6), ethanol. These observations indicate that drug is highly lipophilic in nature. These observations were further confirmed by measurement of partition coefficient of Cephalexin n-Octanol: disitilled water and in n octanol:PBS (pH5.6). The log P in n-Octanol: disitilled water and in n octanol:PBS (pH5.6) were respectively (6.24±0.264) and (6.56±0.018). It shows that the drug is lipophilic in nature. Melting point of Cephalexin was found to be 319±2°C.

All the above observations confirm the identity of Cephalexin. Standard curves of Cephalexin were prepared in methanol and PBS (pH 5.6). The equations of straight line were given in Table 3.5, 3.6 & figure 3.5 and 3.6, respectively. All the curves were found to be linear and correlation coefficient was found to be close to one and found to obey Beer's Lamberts law in the concentration range of 2-20 µg/mL in all cases.

The absorption maxima of drug Cephalexin in methanol (with 2mLDMF) was found to be 268nm. Further compatibility of the drug with phosphatidyl choline (PC), and glyceryl tristearin was observed by determining UV maxima and found to be no significant change in absorption maxima. Thus drug is compatible with these ingredients in the formulation.

Linearity- The response for the drugs was found to be linear in the concentration range 500–1500 ng / spot with correlation co-efficient of 0.9991.

*Analysis of marketed formulation-*A single spot at Rf 0.56 was observed in the chromatogram of the drug samples extracted from tablets. There was no interference from the excipients present in the tablets. The drug content was found to be 102.90 %.

Acidic hydrolytic condition- Cephalexin degrades to considerable extent with acidic hydrolysis. On heating at 80 °C in 0.1 N HCl (1 hour), the height of the drug peak decreased, with corresponding appearance of new degradation peaks. One peak of the degradation product was observed (D1 Rf = 0.76) (Figure- 3.4).

*Alkaline hydrolytic condition-*Cephalexin also degrades rapidly with alkaline hydrolysis. On treatment with 0.01 N NaOH for 1/2 hour, the height of peak was reduced and four new peaks of degradation products were observed (D2

Rf = 0.15, D3 Rf = 0.62, D4 Rf = 0.78 and D5 Rf = 0.82) (Figure – 3.5).

Oxidative condition- Cephalexin was found to degrade less rapidly in oxidative conditions. Upon treatment with 30 % hydrogen peroxide at room temperature for three days, peak height was reduced, with the appearance of one new degradation peak. (D7 Rf = 0.73) (Figure - X)

Dry heat and Photolytic studie- Under dry heat (Oven, 800 C, 12 hour) and photolytic studies, no additional peaks were observed and drug peak area remained constant. This indicates stability of drugs in dry heat, UV light and fluorescent light for specified period.

Chapter-4

Result & Discussion

4.1 Formula:

Table	4.1 Composition of agglomerates			
Materials	Formulation-1	Formulation-2	Formulation-3	Formulation-4
Cephalexin	375mg	375mg	375mg	375mg
Hydroxy Propyl methylCellulose (HPMC) 15 cps	35 mg	42.3mg	-	-
Urdragit L-100	-	-	27.3mg	19.8 mg
Lactose	40 mg	32.7 mg	47.7 mg	55.2 mg
Mg.sterate	5 mg	5mg	5 mg	5 mg

4.2 Evaluation of Powder:

Product	Batch 1(gm)	Batch 2(gm)	Batch 3(gm)	Batch 4(gm)
Mass	50	50	50	50
Volume	78	79	78	76
After 500 tapping	62	64	63	63
After 750 tapping	62	64	63	63

4.3 Average weight of tablet

Batch 1 (mg)	Batch 2(mg)	Batch 3(mg)	Batch 4(mg)	Parameter
0.455	0.455	0.454	0.453	Average weight
0.460	0.460	0.459	0.461	Maximum weight
0.448	0.449	0.447	0.448	Minimum weight
9.068	9.057	8.530	9.007	Initial weight
9.068	9.09	9.075	9.053	Final weight
0.29	0.36	0 .6	0.5	Friability
10-14 KP	10-14 KP	10-14 KP	10-14 KP	Hardness
4.0-4.3	4.0-4.3	4.0-4.3	4.0-4.3	Thickness

4.4 Bulk density of raw material

Product	Batch 1	Batch 2	Batch 3	Batch 4
Bulk density (f0) Mass/volume	50/78 = 0.641	50/79 = 0.632	50/78 = 0.641	50/76 = 0.657
Tapped tansity (ft) Mass/tap.vol.	50/62 =0.806	54/64 = 0.781	50/63 = 0.794	50/63 = 0.79
Hausner's ratio(ft/fo)	0.806/0.641 =1.25	0.781/0.632 =1.23	0.794/0.641 = 1.23	0.79/0.657 = 1.20
Car's complesibility index(ft-fo/ft .100)	20.47 (Fair possable)	19.0 (Fair possable)	19.26 (Fair possable)	16.83 (Good)

4.5 Description of instrument/ equipment

S.No.	Name of the Instrument	Qualified
1.	Friability tester	Yes
2.	Hardness tester	Yes
3.	Disintegration apparatus	Yes
4.	Dissolution apparatus	Yes
5.	Weighing balance	Yes
6.	U.V. apparatus	Yes
7.	F.T.I.R. apparatus	Yes

1. **Tablet Hardness Tester**

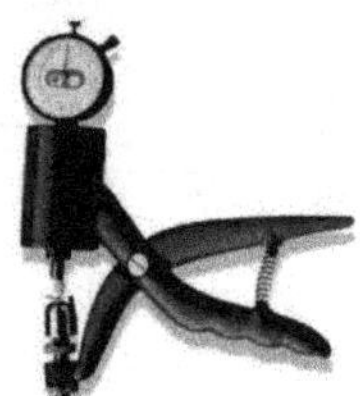

Model	CTHT
capacity	20 Kgs.
Max. Tablet Dia.	25 mm
Net weight (Approx.)	1 Kg.
Gross weight (Approx.)	2.2 Kgs.
Machine Dimensions	410 (L) x 680 (B)

Case Dimension	30.5 (L) x 25.5 (B) x 7.5 (H)

2. **Tablet Disintegration Test Appratus**

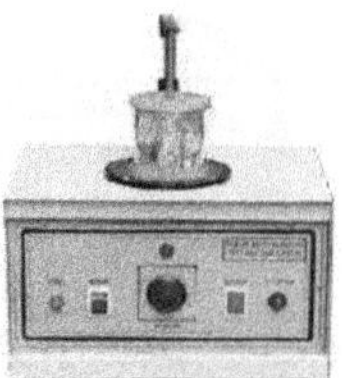

(As per I.P. Third edition 1985) Available in SINGLE BASKET ,TWO BASKET, FOUR BASKET Used for determination of disintegration of time of Tablets. The test equipment consist of 1 litre Beaker, tablet can be tested simultaneously through motorized shaft moves up and down direction of 28 to 32 R.P.M approx.; carrying a rigid basket rack assembly. On the upper end of the shaft is fitted a horizontal strip to support cylindrical standard size glass tubes with stainless steel wire gauge bottom. Cylindrical basket moves up and down with standard perforated made of acrylic sheet inside in one litre glass beaker of distilled water. Unit having hot plate rating 65 watts fixed on the top for BEAKER . Temperature can be maintained by thermostat in between 35 C to 37 C . Digital timer can be fixed with the machine.

3 Friability test apparatus

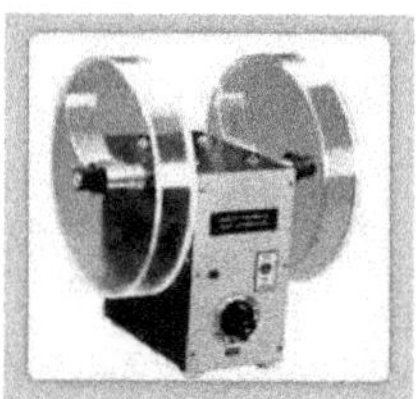

This machine is specially to determine the durability of tablets from the time of production to the time use, as its is important to test abrasion and impact hardness of the tablets. The apparatus consist of transparent acrylic drums. The drums are equipped with a plastic blade which carries the tablets along with it upto predetermined height while the drums are rotating and tablets are allowed to slide and let them slide down. The tablets are weight before and after the rubbing in the drum have taken place. The difference in weight indicates the rate of abrasion.

The microprocessor fabricator is equipped with Micro-Computer based Digital display system. The touch switches are provided on the front panel of the apparatus for setting the required total number of revolution of the drum which rotates at 25 revolutions per minute. Each revolution of the from starting from minimum number 1 to required set number to 9999 is displayed on the window as per pre-setting. An audible alarm sounds alarming the operator that the test over. In this new sophisticated model calculator is not required, as the percentage of the abrasion of the tablets is directly displayed on the front panel by feeding the correct data with the help of programmable touch Switches.

Speed :	25 RPM
Accuracy :	1 RPM
Counter :	1 to 9999 revolutions
No. of Drums :	One or Two as per model
Display :	4 Digits LED

Dimensions: 26 cm x 20 cm x 25 cm

Supply :   230 V / 50 Hz 1 Ph.
(Optional 110 V 60 Hz)

4 Table compression machine (Single rotatory)

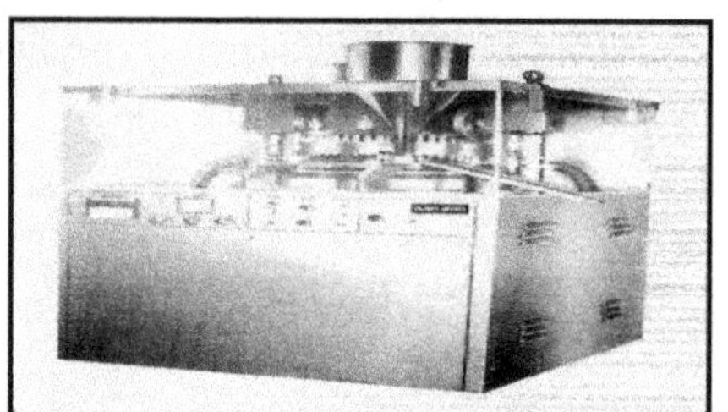

Single Rotary Compression Machine (CLIT

Jamsekey CM 84):

Specification	No. of punch 16
Capacity	70 tablet\rotation
Speed	Max. 36 min. 24
Capacity	Max. 1500 Tab\min.

4.6 Direct Compression:

These are few crystalline substance such Lactose, Mg.Sterate, HPMC15CPS, EUDRAGIT, CEPHALEXIN may be compressed directly. In Directly compressible diluents is an inert substance that may be compactd with little difficulty and may compress even when quantities of drug are mixed with it compression capacity is still maintaind when other tablet materials necessary for flow .

4.7 Step:

- Raw Material

- Weight R.M.

- Shifting

- Mixing

- Shifting

- Mixing

- Compression

4.8 Raw Material:

Check the raw material Quantities. As per the quantity design by the formula or experimental plan. And prepare the lable and affixed on the polybag.

4.9 Weighing:

Weigh the ingredient by the help of weighing balance as per the formula design and separate in the polybag

4.10 Shifting and Mixing:

Shift the ingredient one by one through the mechanical shifter, The granules required for batch 4 (4000 tablets) were prepared by direct granulation technique) as per the formula .

The drug and HPMC and EUDRAGIT an were separately passed through sieve #40 and 60, respectively and mixed with lactose, which was previously passed throughsieve #40, in a double cone blender.ultimately obtained granules were lubricated with magnesium stearate bymixing in Octagonal blendar,(cadmach Engineers, India) at slow speedfor 5 min .

4.11 Compression:

Were compressed to tablets by using 15/32 flat punche by using validated 16station compression machine using single punch.(clit jamesky engineering,Italy) To study the effect of hardness on release profile, in each batchthree sub-batches 1, 2,3 and 4were prepared with hardness of 6—8, 8—1010—12 and 12-14 kg/cm2, respectively.

5. Evaluation:-

5.1 Hardness test:

The crushing strength (Kg/cm²) tablets was determined by using Monosanto hardness tester. In all the cases, means of six replicate determinations were taken. The results are given in table 4.3

5.2 Friability test:

This was determined by weighing 10 tablets after dusting, placing them in the friabilator and rotating the plastic cylinder vertically at 25 rpm for 4 min. After dusting, the total remaining weight of the tablets was recorded

5.3 Uniformity of weight:

The weight (mg) of each of 20 individual tablets was determined by dusting each tablet off and placing it in an electronic balance[78]. The weight data from the tablets were analyzed for sample mean and percent deviation. The results are summarized table 4.3

5.4 Uniformity of drug content:

5 tablets were powdered in a glass mortar and the powder equivalent to 50 mg of drug was placed in a stoppered 100 ml conical flask. The drug was extracted with 40 ml methanol with vigorous shaking on a mechanical gyratory shaker (100 rpm) for 1 hour. Then heated on water bath with occasional shaking for 30 minutes and filtered into 50 ml volumetric flask through cotton wool and filtrate was made up to the mark by passing more methanol through filter, further appropriate dilution were made and absorbance was measured at 225.3nm against blank (methanol).

5.5 In Vitro Dissolution Studies:

In vitro dissolution studies of HBS of Cephalexin were carried out in USPXXIII tablet dissolution test apparatus-II (Electrolab), employing a paddle stirrer at 50 rpm using 900ml of 0.1N HCl at 37±0.5°C as dissolution medium. One tablet was used in each test. At predetermined time intervals 5ml of the samples were withdrawn by means of a syringe fitted with pre filter. The volume withdrawn at each interval was replaced with same quantity of fresh dissolution medium maintained at 37±0.5°C. The samples were analyzed for drug release by measuring the absorbance at 224.6nm using UV-Visible spectrophotometer after suitable dilutions. All the studies were conducted in triplicate.

The results of *in vitro* release profiles obtained for all the formulations were fitted into four models of data treatment as follows:

1. Cumulative percent drug released versus time (zero-order kinetic model).
2. Log cumulative percent drug remaining versus time. (first-order kinetic model).
3. Cumulative percent drug released versus square root of time (Higuchi's model).
4. Log cumulative percent drug released versus log time (Korsmeyer-Peppas equation).

1. Zero Order Kinetics:

A zero-order release would be predicted by the following equation.

$$A_t = A_0 - K_0 t \dots 1$$

Where:

A_t = Drug release at time 't'

A_0 = Initial drug concentration

K_0 = Zero-order rate constant (hr^{-1}).

When the data is plotted as cumulative percent drug release versus time, if the plot is linear then the data obeys zero-order release kinetics, with a slope equal to K_0.

2. First Order Kinetics:

A first-order release would be predicted by the following equation

$$\text{Log } C = \text{Log } C_0 - \dots 2$$

Where:

C = Amount of drug remained at time 't'

C_0 = Initial amount of drug

K = First-order rate constant (hr^{-1}).

When the data is plotted as log cumulative percent drug remaining versus time yields a straight line, indicating that the release follows First-order kinetics.

The constant 'K' can be obtained by multiplying 2.303 with slope values.

3. Higuchi's Model:

Drug released from the matrix devices by diffusion has been described by following Higuchi's classical diffusion equation.

$$Q = \quad \ldots 3$$

Where:

Q = Amount of drug released at time 't'

D = Diffusion coefficient of the drug in the matrix

A = Total amount of drug in unit volume of matrix

C_s = The solubility of the drug in the diffusion medium

ε = Porosity of the matrix

τ = Tortuosity

t = Time (hrs) at which 'Q' amount of drug is released.

Equation-3 may be simplified if one assumes that D, C_s and A are constant. Then equation-3 becomes:

$$Q = Kt^{1/2} \quad \ldots 4$$

When the data is plotted according to equation-4 i.e., cumulative drug released versus square root of time, yields a straight line, indicating that the drug was released by diffusion mechanism[79]. The slope is equal to 'K'.

4. Korsmeyer and Peppas Model:

The release rates from controlled release polymeric matrices can be described by the equation (5) proposed by korsmeyer et al[80].

$$Q = K_1 t^n \ \dots\ 5$$

Q is the percentage of drug released at time 't', K is a kinetic constant incorporating structural and geometric characteristics of the tablets and 'n' is the diffusional exponent indicative of the release mechanism[81].For Fickian release, n=0.45 while for anomalous (Non-Fickian) transport, n ranges between 0.45 and 0.89 and for zero order release, $n = 0.89$[80].

In Vitro Drug Release Data of Trial Formulation T1

Sl. No.	Time (Hrs)	Square Root of Time	Log Time	Cumulative* Percentage Drug Release±SD	Log Cumulative Percentage Drug Release	Cumulative Percent Drug Remaining	Log cumulative Percent Drug Remaining
1	1	1.0000	0.0000	15.72±0.16	1.1965	84.28	1.9257
2	2	1.4142	0.3010	23.94±0.07	1.3791	76.06	1.8812
3	3	1.7320	0.4771	36.70±0.28	1.5647	63.30	1.8014
4	4	2.0000	0.6021	39.82±0.28	1.6001	60.18	1.7795
5	5	2.2360	0.6990	50.63±0.27	1.7044	49.37	1.6935
6	6	2.4494	0.7782	60.01±0.16	1.7782	39.99	1.6020
7	7	2.6457	0.8451	68.31±0.28	1.8345	31.69	1.5009
8	8	2.8284	0.9031	72.50±0.27	1.8603	27.50	1.4393
9	9	3.0000	0.9542	74.82±0.39	1.8740	25.18	1.4011
10	10	3.1622	1.0000	76.44±0.29	1.8833	23.56	1.3722

In vitro drug release data of trial formulation T2

Sl. No.	Time (Hrs)	Square Root of Time	Log Time	Cumulative* Percentage Drug Release±SD	Log Cumulative Percentage Drug Release	Cumulative Percent Drug Remaining	Log cumulative Percent Drug Remaining
1	1	1.0000	0.0000	16.39±0.09	1.2146	83.61	1.9223
2	2	1.4142	0.3010	45.14±0.51	1.6546	54.86	1.7393
3	3	1.7320	0.4771	46.20±0.08	1.6646	53.80	1.7308
4	4	2.0000	0.6021	46.50±0.44	1.6675	53.50	1.7284
5	5	2.2360	0.6990	48.01±0.36	1.6813	51.99	1.7159
6	6	2.4494	0.7782	60.70±0.29	1.7832	39.30	1.5944
7	7	2.6457	0.8451	64.04±0.20	1.8065	35.96	1.5558
8	8	2.8284	0.9031	66.59±0.27	1.8234	33.41	1.5239
9	9	3.0000	0.9542	70.45±0.14	1.8479	29.55	1.4706
10	10	3.1622	1.0000	72.67±0.29	1.8614	27.33	1.4366

In vitro drug release data of trial formulation T3

Sl. No.	Time (Hrs)	Square Root of Time	Log Time	Cumulative* Percentage Drug Release±SD	Log Cumulative Percentage Drug Release	Cumulative Percent Drug Remaining	Log cumulative Percent Drug Remaining
1	1	1.0000	0.0000	6.79±0.13	0.8319	93.21	1.9695
2	2	1.4142	0.3010	12.99±0.07	1.1136	87.01	1.9396
3	3	1.7320	0.4771	24.46±0.14	1.3885	75.54	1.8782
4	4	2.0000	0.6021	38.72±0.27	1.5879	61.28	1.7873
5	5	2.2360	0.6990	46.11±0.05	1.6638	53.89	1.7315
6	6	2.4494	0.7782	54.47±0.27	1.7362	45.53	1.6583
7	7	2.6457	0.8451	59.88±0.27	1.7773	40.12	1.6034
8	8	2.8284	0.9031	63.08±0.28	1.7999	36.92	1.5673
9	9	3.0000	0.9542	64.82±0.28	1.8117	35.18	1.5463
10	10	3.1622	1.0000	67.19±0.21	1.8273	32.81	1.5160

Cumulative Percent Drug Released Vs Time Plots
(Zero Order) of formulations T1, T2 and T3

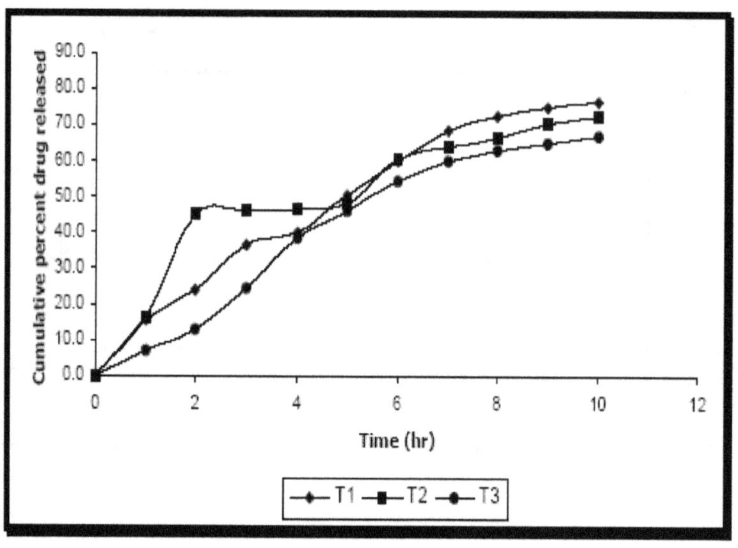

Log Cumulative Percent Drug Remaining Vs Time
Plots (First Order) of
Formulations T1, T2 and T3

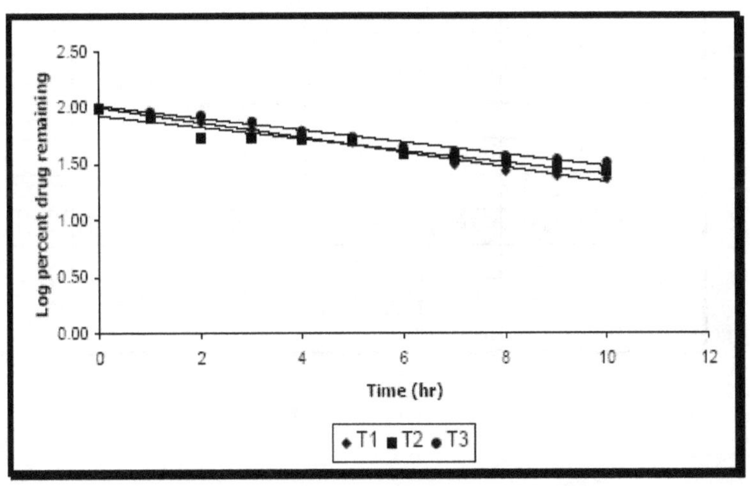

In Vitro Drug Release Data of Trial Formulation T4

Sl. No.	Time (Hrs)	Square Root of Time	Log Time	Cumulative* Percentage Drug Release±SD	Log Cumulative Percentage Drug Release	Cumulative Percent Drug Remaining	Log cumulative Percent Drug Remaining
1	1	1.0000	0.0000	23.48±0.04	1.3707	76.52	1.8838
2	2	1.4142	0.3010	59.23±0.21	1.7725	40.77	1.6103
3	3	1.7320	0.4771	63.06±0.21	1.7998	36.94	1.5675
4	4	2.0000	0.6021	66.99±0.91	1.8260	33.01	1.5186
5	5	2.2360	0.6990	70.20±0.34	1.8463	29.80	1.4742
6	6	2.4494	0.7782	76.42±0.35	1.8832	23.58	1.3725
7	7	2.6457	0.8451	78.93±0.34	1.8972	21.07	1.3237
8	8	2.8284	0.9031	81.00±0.40	1.9085	19.00	1.2788
9	9	3.0000	0.9542	84.81±0.45	1.9284	15.19	1.1816
10	10	3.1622	1.0000	95.21±0.27	1.9787	4.79	0.6803

Cumulative Percent Drug Released vs Time Plots Of
Formulations t4,

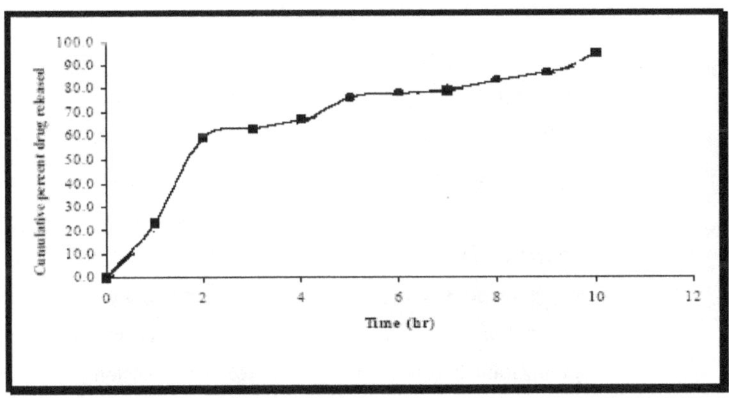

Chapter-5

Methodology & Evaluation

Discussion

In the present study, Extended release tablets of Cephalexin were prepared by using different viscosity grades of hydroxy propyl methyl cellulose (HPMC) viz.,Eudragit and 50 cps, at different drug to polymer

The prepared Extended tablets were evaluated for hardness, friability, uniformity of weight, uniformity of drug content, swelling index, *in vitro* dissolution, short-term stability and drug-polymer interaction. Formulation optimization has been done by Direct compression then evaluating the preliminary data obtained from four batches of formulations (T_1 to T_4).

The hardness of the prepared Extended release tablet was found to be in the range of 10 -14 Kg/cm². The friability of all tablets was less than 1% i.e., in the range of 0.29 to 0.61%. The percentage deviation from the mean weights of all the batches of prepared tablets were found to be within the prescribed limits as per IP. The low values of standard deviation indicates uniform drug content in all the batches prepared as observed from the data given in table.

In vitro floating studies were performed by placing tablets in USP XXIII dissolution the apparatus-II containing 900 ml of 0.1N HCl maintained at a temperature of 37±0.5°C. The results are given in tables-9 & 10. For all formulations.

In vitro drug release study was performed using USP XXIII dissolution test apparatus-II at 50 rpm using 900 ml of 0.1N HCl maintained at 37±0.5°C as the dissolution medium. The results were shown in tables-**11 to 25.** From the above data, it is evident that as the proportion of polymer in the formulation increases, cumulative percent drug release in 10 hours decreases, and as the proportion of the EUDRAGIT increases, the drug release Increases

Among the four trial batches, formulations T1 and T2 have released only 67 to 76% drug in 10 hours, whereas formulations T3 and T4 have released 81 to 95% during the same period. This increased drug release from these formulations can be attributed to the lower viscosity grade (50 cps) of HPMC

It was found that in comparative invitro study of prepared tablet and a marketed product **(Phexin- BD375 mg)** total percentage drug release over 24hrs. was range from 67 to 76% of t1 and t2 batches respectively and 81 to 95% of t3 and t4 respectively therefore maeketed product shown lesser percentage drug release profile than t4 batch.

Phexin-BD 375 mg:

Phexin- BD is a extended release oral formulation of cephalexin designed to be effective on twice daily dosing. Cephalexin is a semisynthetic Cephalosporin antibiotic intended for administration.

Molecular Formula: $C_{16}H_{17}N_3O_4S \cdot H_2O$

Molecular Weight: 347.393

Structure formula:

The nucleus of cephlexin is releated to that of other cephalosporin antibiotic.The compound is a zwitterion i.e. the molecule both a basic and an acidic group.The isoelectric point of cephalexin in water is approximately 4.5 to 5.The crystalline from of cephalexin which is available is a monohydrate. It is a white crystalline solid having a bitter taste. Solubility in water is low at room temperature; 1or 2 mg/ml may be dissolved readily,but higher concentration are obtained with increasing difficulity.The cephalosporins differ from penicillins in the bicyclic ring system. Cephalexin has a D- phenylglycyl group as substituent at the 7-amino position and an unsubstituted methyl group at the 3-postion.

Manufacturer: Glaxosmithkline Ltd.

Chapter-6

Summary & Conclusion

The formulation of Cephalexin tablet and evaluation. As a main objectives evidence that a process consistently produce a product that are suitable for their intended use. To watch out the critical steps of manufacturing of Cephalexin formulation is key element assuring that these principles and goals are met.

In this study of formulation and evaluation of Cephalexin tablet was carried out as solid dosage form. Critical parameters were taken up:

➢ Granulation
➢ Blending
➢ Compression
➢ Packing

As the formulation completed, even in process the evaluation of tablet which would be conducted some important evaluation as:

- Content Uniformity Test for Tablets

- Mechanical strength of tablets

- Friability Test for Tablets

- Hardness or Crushing strength of Tablets

- Tensile strength

- Brittle fracture index (BFI)

- Tablet Disintegration

- Theories of disintegration of Tablets

- Tablet Dissolution Test

Chapter-7

Reference

1. Qiu, Y. & Zhang, G. (2000). Research and Development Aspects of Oral Controlled Release Systems; *Handbook of Pharmaceutical Controlled Release Technology,* Marcel Dekker, Inc., New York, NY. pp. 465 – 503.

2. Qiu, Y. (2007). Design and Evaluation of Oral Modified-Release Dosage Forms Based on Drug Property and Delivery Technology. Proc. CAE/AAPS/CPA/CRS/FIP/APSTJ Conference: Oral Controlled Release Development and Technology. Shanghai, pp. 34–43.

3. Getsios , D. , Caro , J.J. , Ishak , K.J. , El-Hadi , W. , Payne , K. , O'Connel , M. ,Albrecht , D. , Feng , W. & Dubois , D. (2004) . Oxybutynin extended release and tolterodine immediate release. Clin. Drug Invest. 24 (2), 81 – 88.

4. Guidance for Industry. (1997). SUPAC-MR: Modified Release Solid Oral Dosage Forms Scale-Up and Postapproval Changes: Chemistry, Manufacturing, and Controls; *In vitro* Dissolution Testing and *In vivo* Bioequivalence Documentation. US Department of Health and Human Services, Food and Drug Administration, Center for Drug Evaluation and Research.

5. Wise, D.L., Klibanov, A.M., Langer, R., Mikos, A.G., Peppas, N.A.,

6. Trantolo, D.J. Wnek, G.E. & Yaszeski, M.J. (eds). *Handbook of Pharmaceutical Controlled Release Technology,* Marcel Dekker, Inc., New York, NY.

7. C.M. Amabile, B.J. Bowman, Overview of oral modified-releaseopioid products for the management of chronic pain,Ann. Pharmacother. 40 (2006) 1327–1335.

8. P.J. Wiffen, J.E. Edwards, J. Barden, H.J.M. McQuay, Oral morphine for cancer pain, http://www.cochrane.org (2006).

9. J.R. Caldwell, Avinza-24 h sustained-release oral morphine therapy, Expert Opin. Pharmacother. 5 (2004) 469–472.

10. Spyker, D.A., Thomas, B.L., Sande, M.A., Bolton, W.K., 1978. Pharmacokinetics of cefaclor and cephalexin dosage nomograms for impaired renal function Antimicrob Agents Chemother,14, 172 177.

11. Sweetman, S., 2003. Martindale: The Complete Drug Reference. Sweetman, S. (Ed.), Micromedex, Electronic Version. Pharmaceutical Press, Greenwood Village, Colorado.

12. Williams, D., 2002. pKa Values for Some Drugs and Miscellaneous Organic Acids and Bases., Foye's Principle of Medicinal Chemistry, Edition 5, p. 1071, Lippincott Williams and Wilkins, Philidelphia.

13. Poisindex 2003 Poisindex System. Toll, L.L., Hurlbut, K.M. (Ed.), Micromedex, Electronic

14. Version. Pharmaceutical Press, Greenwood Village, Colorado.

15. AHFS 2001 Drug Monographs. McEvoy, G. (Ed.), American Hospital Formulary System, pp. 128–253,

16. N.A. Peppas, Hydrogels in Medicine, CRS Press, Boca Raton, FL, 1986.

17. F. Alhaique, E. Santucci, M. Carafa, T. Coviello, E. Murtas, F.M. Riccieri, Gellan in sustained release formulations: preparation of gel capsules and release studies, Biomaterials 17 (1996) 1981–1986.

18. M.V. Risbud, R.R. Bhonde, Polyacrylamide-chitosan hydrogels: in vitro biocompatibility and sustained

19. antibiotic release studies, Drug Deliv. 7 (2000) 69–75.

20. K.S. Soppimath, T.M. Aminabhavi, A.M. Dave, S.G. Kumbar, W.E. Rudzinski, Stimulus-responsive smart hydrogels as novel drug delivery systems, Drug Dev. Ind. Pharm. 28 (2002) 957–974.

21. Thornhill T. S., Levison M. E., Johnson W. E., Kaye D., *Appl. Micro Microbiol.*, **17**, 457—461 (1969).

22. Colin D. (ed.), "Therapeutic Drugs," 2nd ed., Churchill Livingstone, Edinburgh, United Kingdom, 1999, pp. c144—c146.

23. Shin S. C., Cho S. J., *Drug Dev. Ind. Pharm.*, **22**, 299—305 (1996).

24. Martinez-Pacheco R., Vila-Jato J. L., Concherio A., Souto C., Ramos T., *Int. J. Pharmaceut.*, **47**, 37—42 (1988).

25. Banker G. S., Anderson N. R., "Theory and Practice of Industrial Pharmacy," 3rd ed., ed. by Lachman L., Lieberman H. A., Kanig J. L., Varghese Publishing House, Mumbai, 1987, pp. 296—329.

26. United States Pharmacopoeia 23, United States Pharmacopoeial Convention, INC., 1995, p. 323.

27. Costa P., Sousa Lobo J. M., *E. J. Pharm. Sci.*, **13**, 123—133 (2001).

28. Nichols W. K., "Anti-infectives, in Remington: The Science and Practice of Pharmacy," 19th ed., ed. by Gennaro A. R., Mack Publishing Company, Pennsylvania, 1995, pp. 1290—1297.

29. Simmons R. J., *Anal. Microbiology*, **II**, 193—195 (1972).

30. Wick W. E., *Applied Microbiology*, **15**, 765—766 (1967)

31. Mitchell K., Ford J. L., *Int. J. Pharmaceut.*, **100**, 175—
179 (1993).

32. Frydman M.A, Chapelle P. Diekmann H.
"Pharmacokinetics of Diltiazem." *Am J Cardiol.*
1989:20:25 33.

33. O'Connor S.E., Grosset A. Janiak P. "The
pharmacological basis and pathophysiological
significance of the heart rate-lowering property of
Diltiazem." Fundamental and Clinical Pharmacology.
1999:13(2):145 53.

34. Sajid M.S, Rimple J., Cheek E. Baig M.K. "The
efficacy of Diltiazem and glyceryltrinitrate for the
medical management of chronic anal fissure: a meta-
analysis". *Int J Colorectal Disease.* 2008:23(1):1-6.

35. Nash GF, Kapoor K, Saeb-Parsy K, Kunanadam T.
Dawson P.M. The long-term results of
Diltiazem treatment for anal fissure. *Int J Cl. Prac.*
2006:60(11):1411-3.

36. Tripathi KD, Essentials of Medical Pharmacology 5th
edition 2003: Jaypee brothers medical Publishers.
New Delhi 488-496.

37. Lachman L, Liberman HA, Kanig JL, The Theory and Practice of Industrial Pharmacy. Mumbai, India: Varghese Publishing House: 1987:430-456.

38. Cooper J.Gunn C. Powder flow and compaction. In: Carter SJ, eds. Tutorial Pharmacy. New Delhi, India: CBS Publishers and Distributors: 1986:211-233.

39. Lachman L.,Lieberman H.A.Kanig J.L.Tablets in The theory and practice of pharmacy Varghese Publishing house 1987:317-320.

40. Shah D, Shah Y, Rampradhan M, Development and evaluation of controlled release Diltiazem hydrochloride microparticles using cross-linked poly(vinyl alcohol). *Drug Del Ind Pharm.* 1997:23(6):567-574.

41. Aulton ME, Wells TI, Pharmaceutics: The Science of Dosage Form Design. London, England: Churchill Livingstone: 1988: 185-189.

42. Martin A, Micromeritics. In: Martin A, eds. Physical Pharmacy. Baltimore, MD: Lippincott Williams & Wilkins: 2001:423-454.

43. Pharmacopoeia of India. New Delhi: Ministry of Health and Family Welfare, Government of India, Controller of Publications : 1996:899-900

44. Lachman L, Liberman HA, Kanig JL, eds. The Theory and Practice of Industrial Pharmacy. Mumbai, India: Varghese Publishing House: 1987:293-345.

45. Aulton ME, Wells TI, Pharmaceutics: The Science of Dosage Form Design. London, England: Churchill Livingstone: 1988:182-183

46. Khemariya P, Bhargava M, Singhai SK, "Preparation and evaluation of mouth dissolving tablets of meloxicam" *Int J Drug Del* 2010:71-78

47. Mutalik S, Hiremath D, Formulation and evaluation of chitosan matrix tablets of nifedipine. The Eastern Pharmacist. 2000:2:109-111.

48. Khan KA, Rhodes CT, Evaluation of different viscosity grades of sodium carboxy methylcellulose as tablet disintegrants. *Pharm Acta Helv*. 1975:50:99-102.

49. Shah NH, Lazarus JH, Jarwoski CL, Carboxy methylcellulose: Effect of degree of polymerization

and substitution on tablet disintegration and dissolution. *J Pharm Sci.* 1981:70 (6):611-613.

50. Korsmeyer RW, Gurny R, Peppas NA, Mechanisms of solute release from porous hydrophilic polymers. *Int J Pharm.* 1983:15:25-35.

51. Fassihi RA, Ritschel WA, Multiple layer, direct compression controlled release system: *In vitro and in vivo* evaluation. *J Pharm Sci.* 1993:82:750- 754.

52. Thornhill T. S., Levison M. E., Johnson W. E., Kaye D., *Applied Microbiology*, 17, 457—461 (1969).

53. Colin Dollery (ed.), "Therapeutic Drugs," 2nd ed., Churchill Livingstone, Edinburgh, 1999, pp. c144 c146.

54. Shin S. C., Cho S. J., *Drug Dev. Ind. Pharm.*, 22, 299—305 (1996).

55. Martinez-Pacheco R., Vila-Jato J. L., Concherio A., Souto C., Ramos T., *Int. J. Pharmaceut.*, 47, 37—42 (1988).

56. Martinez-Pacheco R., Vila-Jato J. L., Souto C., Ramos T., *Int. J. Pharmaceut.* 32, 99—102 (1986).

57. Schneider H., Nightingale C. H., Quintiliani R., Flanagan D. R., *J. Pharm. Sci.*, 67, 1620—1622 (1978).

58. Dhopeshwarkar V., O'Keefe J. C., Zatz J. L., Deeter R., Horton M., *Drug Dev. Ind. Pharm.*, 20, 18511867 (1994).

59. Saravanan M., Nataraj K. S., Ganesh K. S., *Biol. Pharm. Bull.*, 25, 541— 545 (2002).

60. Banker G. S., Anderson N. R., "Theory and Practice of Industrial Pharmacy," 3rd ed., ed. by Lachman L., Lieberman H. A., Kanig J. L., Varghese Publishing House, Mumbai, 1987, pp. 296—329.

61. United States Pharmacopoeia 23 United States Pharmacopoeial Convention, INC., 1995, p. 323.

62. Costa P., Sousa Lobo J. M., *E. J. Pharm. Sci.*, 13, 123—133 (2001).

63. Nichols W. K., "Anti-infectives, in Remington: The Science and Practice of Pharmacy," 19th ed., edited.by Gennaro A. R., Mack Publishing Company, Pennsylvania, 1995, pp. 1290—1297.

64. Simmons R. J., *Anal. Microbiology*, II, 193—195 (1972).

65. Wick W. E., *Applied Microbiology*, 15, 765—766 (1967).

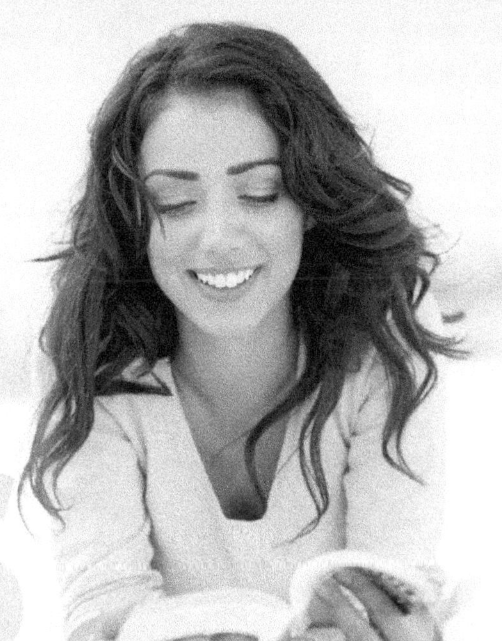

yes i want morebooks!

Buy your books fast and straightforward online - at one of world's fastest growing online book stores! Environmentally sound due to Print-on-Demand technologies.

Buy your books online at
www.get-morebooks.com

Kaufen Sie Ihre Bücher schnell und unkompliziert online – auf einer der am schnellsten wachsenden Buchhandelsplattformen weltweit! Dank Print-On-Demand umwelt- und ressourcenschonend produziert.

Bücher schneller online kaufen
www.morebooks.de

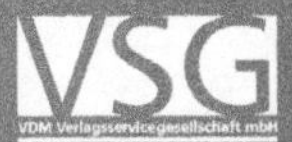

VDM Verlagsservicegesellschaft mbH
Heinrich-Böcking-Str. 6-8   Telefon: +49 681 3720 174   info@vdm-vsg.de
D - 66121 Saarbrücken   Telefax: +49 681 3720 1749   www.vdm-vsg.de